Lotus Illustrated DICTIONARY of MEDICAL

Complied and Edited by.
Hans Baker

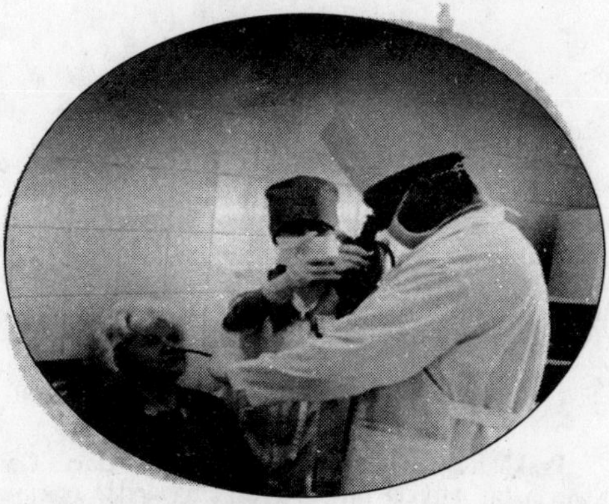

Lotus PRESS
4735/22, Prakash Deep Building
Ansari Road, Daryaganj,
New Delhi - 110002

Lotus Illustrated

DICTIONARY *of* MEDICAL

ISBN 81 89093 49 5

Published by:
Lotus Press Publishers & Distributors
Unit No. 220, 2nd Floor, 4735/22,
Prakash Deep Building, Ansari Road, Darya Ganj,
New Delhi- 110002, Ph.: 32903912, 23280047, 09811838000
• E-mail : lotuspress1984@gmail.com www.lotuspress.co.in

Printed at : Lotus Press Publishers & Distributors, Delhi

PREFACE

Disease is a general term used to refer to any departure from health in which a patient suffers. It can be defined as disorder of bodily function or destructive processes in organs, organs' systems or in an organism with recognisable signs and symptoms, and in many cases a known cause. The words disease, illness and sickness are used often interchangeably but are not synonymous. Rather, whereas disease relates to a physiological or psychological dysfunction, an illness is the subjective state of a patient who feels unwell and sickness encompasses a state of social dysfunction, such as the role that the individual assumes when ill.

The general medicine skill is used to attempt to find out what is wrong with someone who is ill from disease, poisons or something else unspecified. The means to cure almost any disease does exist, but to be effective an accurate diagnoses is required. It is a Hidden Task since a fumbled roll will result in a mis-diagnosis with possibly dangerous results. A diagnosis will take a certain length of time to perform. This will normally be 1-2 hours in a hospital, but with rare causes or less equipment the time will be increased.

Medicine is a substance or combination of substances used or intended to be used to diagnose, treat, mitigate or prevent a disease, disorder or abnormal physical or mental state, or a symptom of them, or to restore, correct or modify organic functions, in man or animal.

It is more strictly, a molecule whose pharmacological activity can be correlated with its chemical structure. Historically, medicines were identified and extracted from naturally occurring fungi, plants, and other flora and fauna, with little direction given to the targeting of a particular disease. Increasingly, however, modern medicines are being discovered through the precise targeting of a particular disease state dissected at the molecular level, and the drugs may be genes, the protein products of genes.

This dictionary explains all type of diseases existing in the world. It also explains different type of chemicals produced in our body and their utilisation for the growth and development.

■ **a.c.**
pharmaceutical abbreviation, before eating (*ante cibum*).

■ **abdomen**
the area of the body between the chest and pelvis, contains the liver, spleen and intestines that are referred to as abdominal organs.

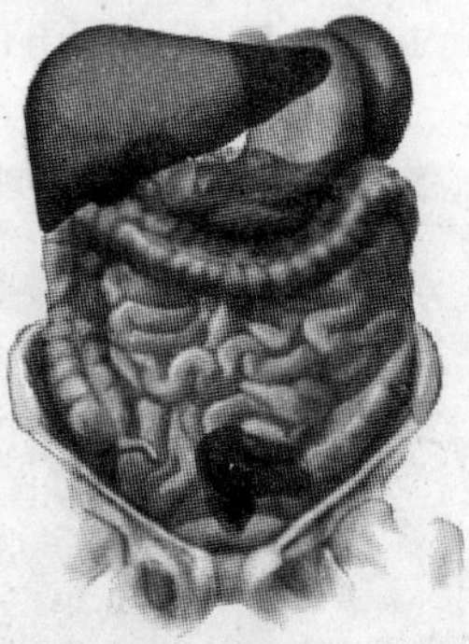

■ **ablation**
surgical removal of a body part.

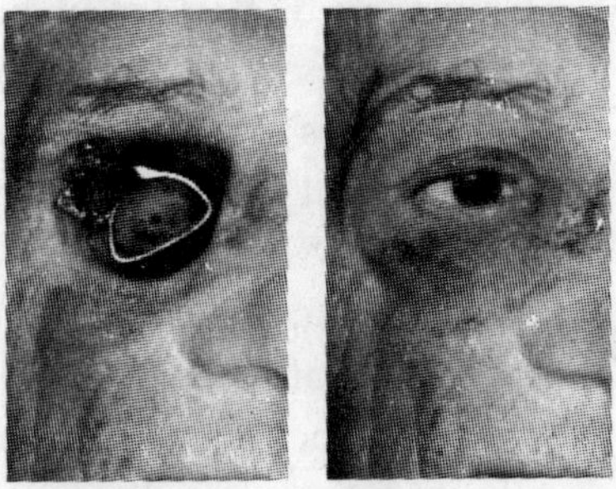

■ **abruption**
tearing away, separation or detachment.

■ **abscess**
an isolated accumulation of pus associated with a localised infection. Abscesses may result in tissue destruction, pain and swelling. Severe abscesses may require surgical drainage.

■ **absolute CD4 cell count**
the number of CD4 cells in a cubic millimetre (mm3) of blood. See also CD4 cell count.

■ **abstract**
a written summary of the important points of a scientific article.

■ **accelerated approval**
FDA regulations, governing early marketing approval of promising drugs for life-threatening illnesses.

■ **Acquired Immunodeficiency Syndrome**
the most severe manifestation of infection with the Human Immunodeficiency Virus (HIV). The Centre for Disease Control and Prevention (CDC) lists numerous opportunistic infections and cancers that, in the presence of HIV infection, constitute an AIDS diagnosis. In 1993, CDC expanded the criteria for an AIDS diagnosis in adults and adolescents to include CD4+ T cell count at or below 200 cells per micro litre, in the presence of HIV infection. In persons (aged 5 and above) with normally functioning im-

mune systems, CD4+ T cell counts usually range from 500-1,500 cells per microlitre. Persons living with AIDS often have infections of the lungs, brain, eyes and other organs and frequently suffer debilitating weight loss, diarrhoea and a type of cancer called Kaposi's Sarcoma.

■ ACTG

abbreviation, AIDS Clinical Trials Group.

■ AACTG

abbreviation, Adult AIDS Clinical Trials Group.

■ ACTG 076

a clinical trial conducted by the ACTG that studied the use of AZT for the reduction of vertical (mother-to-child) transmission of HIV.

■ active immunity

protection from a disease, as a result of previous exposure to the disease-causing infectious agent or antigen. The protection can be a result of having had the disease or having received a vaccine to prevent getting the disease.

■ active immunisation

a process by which a person is inoculated with an antigen to encourage the immune system to mount an immune response, e.g., by producing antibodies.

■ ACTU

abbreviation, AIDS Clinical Testing Unit. Clinical trial sites.

■ acupressure

a method of massage in which pressure is applied to specific acupuncture points with the fingers.

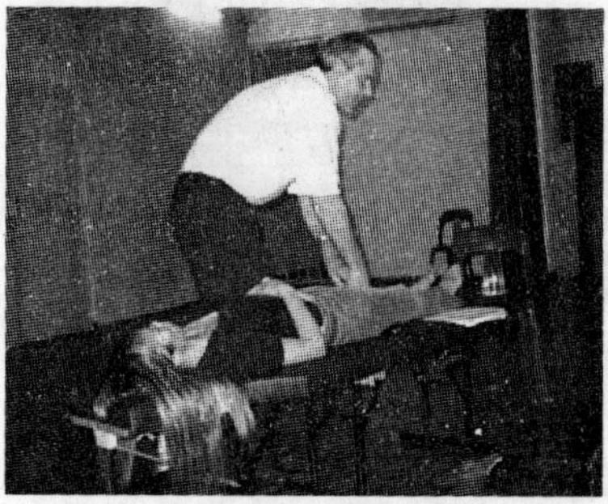

■ acupuncture

a Chinese medical treatment involving the insertion of very fine sterile needles into the body at specific points according to a mapping of 'energy pathways'. Historically, acupuncture is one component of an overall program of Chinese medicine that includes theory, practice, diagnosis, physiology and the use of herbal preparations. Acupuncture is used to control pain and to treat other conditions such as allergies or addiction withdrawal.

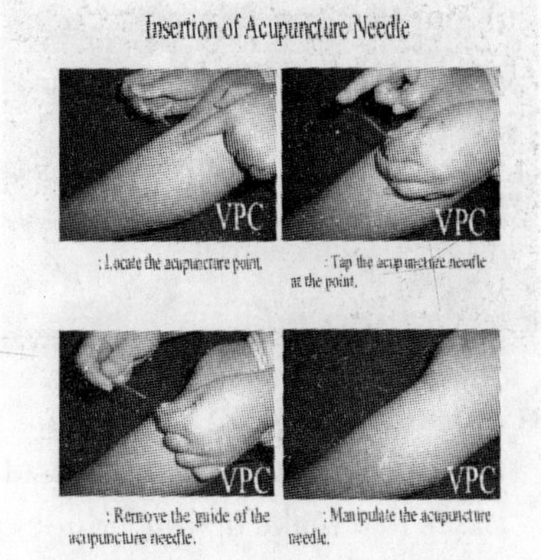

■ **acute**
reaching a crisis quickly.

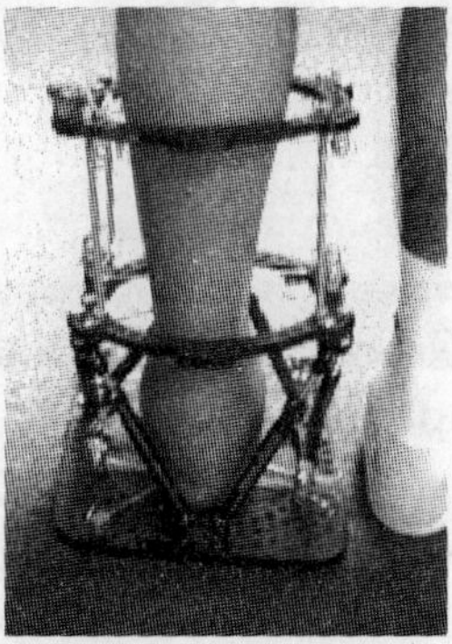

■ **Acute HIV Infection**
the period of rapid viral replication, immediately following exposure to HIV. An estimated 80 to 90 percent of individuals with primary HIV infection develop an acute syndrome characterised by flu-like symptoms of fever, malaise, lymphadenopathy, pharyngitis, headache, myalgia and sometimes rash. Following primary infection, seroconversion and a broad HIV-1 specific immune response occurs, usually within an average of three weeks after transmission of HIV. It was previously thought that HIV was relatively dormant during this phase. However, it is now known that during the time of primary infection, high levels of plasma HIV RNA can be documented.

■ **Acute HIV Infection and Early Diseases Research Program (AIEDRP)**
a program funded by the National Institute of Allergy and Infectious Diseases (NIAID) focusing on innovative ways to study how HIV-1 causes disease in adults. Scientists will use interventions, such as highly active antiretroviral therapy (HAART) given in the acute and early phases of infection, to increase their understanding of the mechanisms and course of HIV disease.

■ **Acute Retroviral Syndrome (ARS)**
a combination of flu-like symptoms, e.g., fever, sore throat, skin rash, headache, nausea, muscle or joint pain that accompanies primary (initial) HIV infection or occurs shortly after the infection. ARS is due to a cellular immune response that takes place before

the immune system has had time to produce antibodies.

■ **acyclovir (zovirax)**

an antiviral drug used to treat herpes simplex virus types 1 and 2 and varicella-zoster virus infections. When used in combination with AZT, acyclovir has been shown in some studies to prolong survival in persons with HIV disease.

■ **ad lib**

pharmaceutical abbreviation, as much as wanted (*ad libitum*).

■ **adaptive immune response**

immune system activation in response to a challenge by a specific pathogen.

■ **ADC**

abbreviation, AIDS Dementia Complex. Deterioration of intellectual faculties often accompanied by emotional disturbances. HIV is active in the brain i.e. central nervous system and can cause dementia, even in those with high CD4 counts and low viral loads. Treatment usually involves an anti-HIV drug, such as AZT, that is able to cross the blood-brain barrier.

■ **addiction**

psychological dependence on a drug.

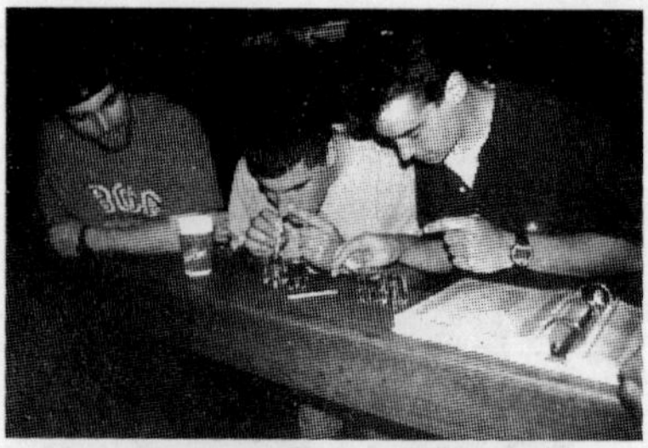

■ **Adenine (A)**

one of the purine nucleic acid bases that make up nucleotides, the building blocks of DNA and RNA. The antiviral drug ddI is a nucleoside analog associated with adenine.

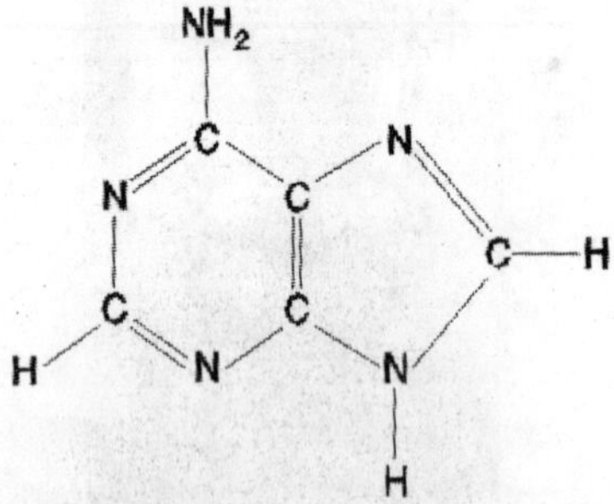

■ **Adeno-Associated Virus (AAV)**

a non-pathogenic virus that may be used as a vector or delivery vehicle in genetic engineering, to insert genes into cells.

■ **adenopathy**

any disease involving or causing enlargement of glandular tissues, especially one involving the lymph nodes.

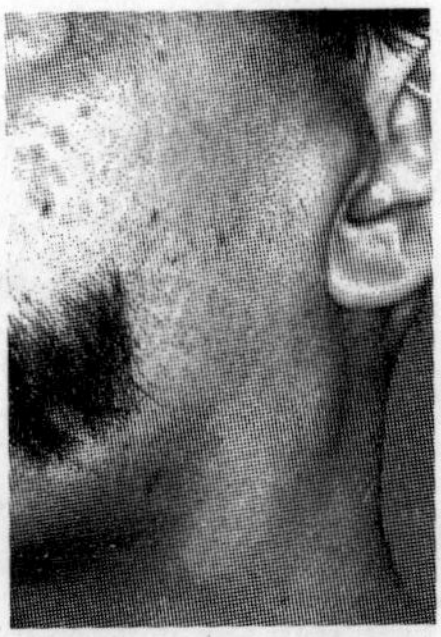

■ **adenovirus**

a family of double-stranded DNA viruses that are the cause of the common cold.

■ **adherence**

the extent to which the patient continues the agreed-upon mode of treatment or intervention as prescribed.

■ **adjunct**

something joined or added to the original. Adjunct therapy or treatment is a treatment that is given in addition to the main or primary treatment.

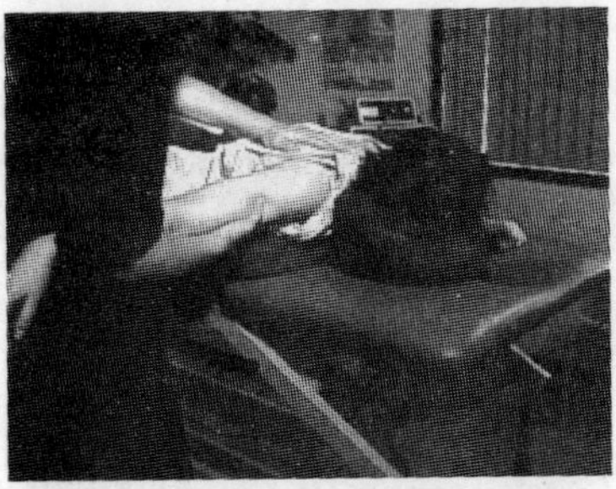

■ **adjuvant**

an ingredient added to a prescription or solution that facilitates or modifies the action of the principal ingredient. May be used in HIV therapies or for HIV vaccines.

■ **adjuvant therapy**

a type of therapy that improves the outcome of a primary therapy, e.g., radiation and chemotherapy are adjuvant therapies in relation to cancer surgery.

■ **administration**

(Route of Administration.) how a drug or therapy is introduced into the body. Systemic administration means that the drug goes throughout the body usually carried in the bloodstream and includes oral, intravenous (injection into the vein, IV), intra-muscular (injection into a muscle, IM), intrathecal (injection into the spinal canal), subcutaneous (injection beneath the skin) and rectal administrations. Local administration means that the drug is applied or introduced into the specific area affected by the disease, such as application directly onto the affected skin surface (topical administration). The effects of most therapies depend upon the ability of the drug to reach the affected area. Thus the route of administration and consequent distribution of a drug in the body are important determinants of its effectiveness.

■ Adoptive Immune Transfer (Adoptive Immunotherapy)

the use of a graft of immune tissue, e.g. bone marrow from a healthy donor to rebuild the immune system in an individual whose immune system has been damaged or destroyed.

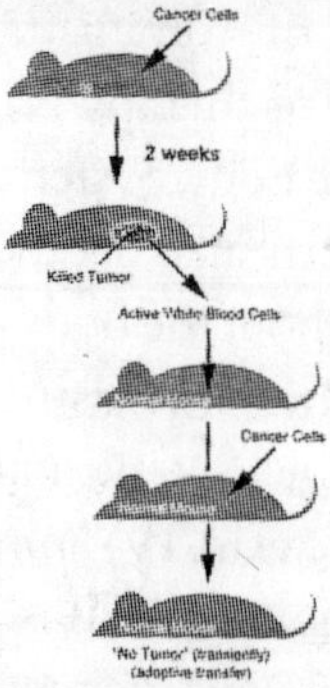

■ adrenal gland

an organ located above each kidney that produces various hormones. The medulla, i.e. the inner part of the adrenal gland secretes adrenaline (epinephrine). The cortex, i.e. the outer part secretes steroids such as cortisol and certain androgens. The adrenal cortex is stimulated to produce hormones by the pituitary hormone ACTH. Reduced secretion (adrenal insufficiency) can lead to fatigue, anorexia and weight loss.

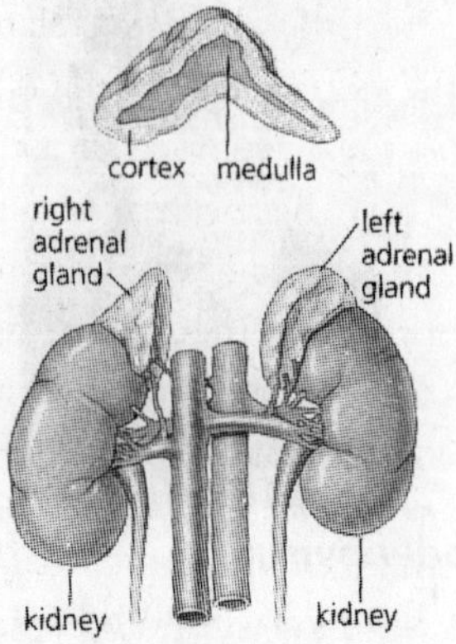

■ adrenaline (epinephrine)

a hormone produced by the cortex of the adrenal gland, particularly during intense emotional states such as fear and rage. Adrenaline increases the heart rate, relaxes bronchial and intestinal smooth muscle and increases certain metabolic processes. Adrenaline is used to treat acute allergic reactions and asthma.

■ Adrenocorticotrophic Hormone (ACTH)

a hormone produced by the pituitary gland to regulate the production of hormones by the adrenal cortex, including cortisol.

■ Adult Aids Clinical Trials Group (AACTG)

the largest HIV clinical trial organisation in the world. It plays a major role in setting standards of care for HIV infection and opportunistic diseases related to HIV/AIDS in the United States and the developed world. The AACTG has been pivotal in providing the data necessary for the approval of therapeutic agents, as well as the treatment and prevention strategies, for many opportunistic infections and prevention strategies, for many opportunistic infections and malignancies. The AACTG is composed of and directed by leading clinical scientists in HIV/AIDS therapeutic research and funded through the National Institute of Allergy and Infectious Diseases.

■ Adverse Experience Report

a form used in clinical trials to document life-threatening toxicities, abbreviated as AER.

■ adverse reaction

side-effect; an undesirable or allergic response to a drug. Many of the drugs used to fight HIV disease cause adverse reactions in a small number of people. Some side effects are minor and others go away after a few days. A few are truly nasty and require quick medical attention. Adverse reactions may range from mild effects such as rash, headache, nausea or drowsiness, to more severe effects such as peripheral neuropathy, bone marrow suppression, seizures and liver or kidney failure.

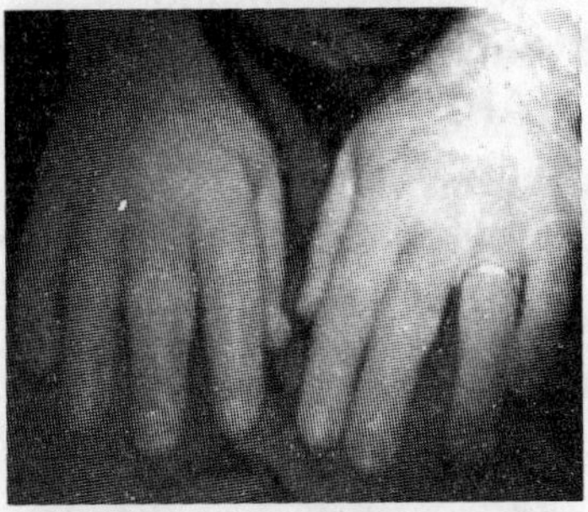

■ aerobic

requiring or living in the presence of oxygen, e.g. aerobic bacteria.

■ aerobic exercise

a type of exercise, e.g. running, swimming, that makes the heart and lungs work harder, to supply the muscles with more oxygen.

■ aerosol

a fine mist, an aerosolised drug is administered as a fine spray that is inhaled into the lungs.

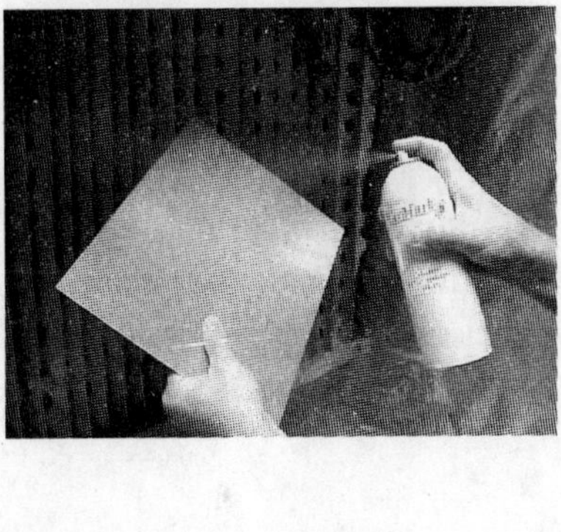

aerosolised
a liquid dispensed as a fine mist or gas which is inhaled, derived from AERO (air) + SOL(solution).

Aerosolised Pentamidine (AP)
a drug inhaled as a fine mist for prophylaxis against Pneumocystis Carinii Pneumonia (PCP).

afebrile
without a fever.

affected community
persons living with HIV and AIDS and other related individuals, including their families, friends and advocates whose lives are directly influenced by HIV infection and its physical, psychological and sociological ramifications.

affective illness
a condition, e.g. depression, mania, that affects the mood.

afferent
refers to nerves that travel from the rest of the body, e.g. skin, muscles organs to the brain and spinal cord..

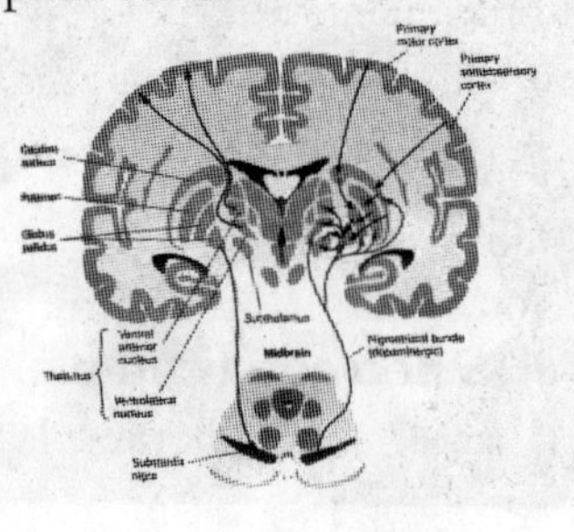

agammaglobulinemia
a nearly total absence of immunoglobulins resulting in the loss of the ability to produce immune antibodies.

Agency For Healthcare Research And Quality (AHRQ)
provides evidence-based information on heath care outcomes, quality, cost, use and access. Information from AHRQ research data, helps people make more informed decisions and improve the quality of health care services. AHRQ was formerly known as the Agency for Health Care Policy and Research

aggressive treatment
a treatment regimen that employs as many useful therapies as possible, even those that are experimental or involve adverse side effects.

agonist
an agent that binds to a receptor on a cell's surface and promotes a specific cellular activity. Agonists often exert their effect by mimicking the activity of the body's natural neurotransmitters and other regulatory chemicals or of other drugs. Also refers to a drug

or substance that promotes the activity of another drug.

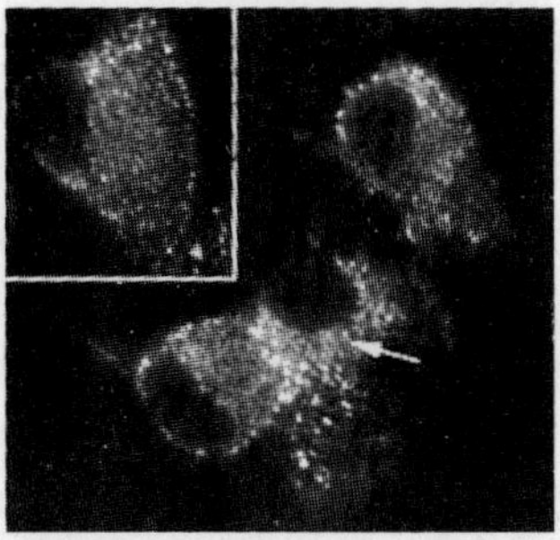

■ **agranulocyte**
a type of white blood cell, e.g. macrophage, lymphocyte that does not contain granules of toxic chemicals.

■ **AIDS**
see **Acquired Immunodeficiency Syndrome**

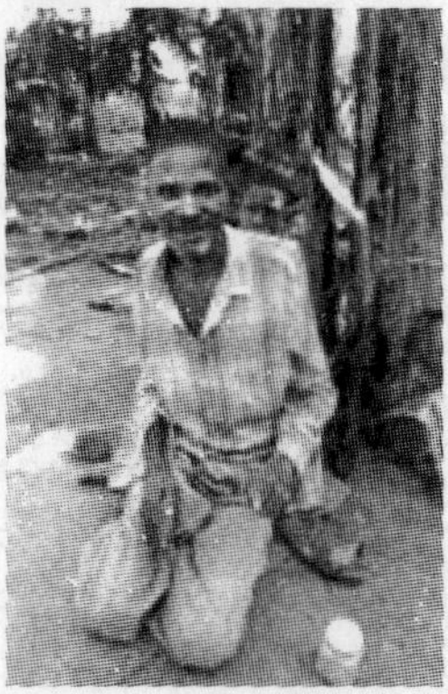

■ **Aids Clinical Trials Information Service (ACTIS)**
provides quick and easy access to information on federally and privately funded clinical trials that evaluate experimental drugs and other therapies for adults and children at all stages of HIV infection. ACTIS is co-sponsored by the Food and Drug Administration, the National Institute of Allergy and Infectious Diseases, the Centre for Disease Control and Prevention and the National Library of Medicine. The HIV/AIDS Clinical Trials Information Service (ACTIS) and its sister service, the HIV/AIDS Treatment Information Service (ATIS), have merged into AIDSinfo. AIDSinfo includes all of the services that were available from ACTIS and ATIS and much more.

■ **AIDS clinical testing unit**
clinical trial sites, commonly abbreviated as ACTU.

■ **AIDS Clinical Trials Group**
federal AIDS drug testing organisation, commonly abbreviated as ACTG.

■ **AIDS-defining illness**
a condition, e.g., Pneumocystis carinii pneumonia, toxoplasmosis, Kaposi's sarcoma that is included in the Centre for Disease Control and Prevention's CDC definition of AIDS.

■ **AIDS dementia complex**
HIV-associated dementia or

HAD. A degenerative neurological condition attributed to HIV infection, characterised by a group of clinical presentations including loss of coordination, mood swings, loss of inhibitions and widespread cognitive dysfunction. It is the most common central nervous system complication of HIV infection. Characteristically, it manifest's itself after the patient develops major opportunistic infections or AIDS-related cancers. However, patients can also have this syndrome before these major systemic complications occur. The cause of ADC has not been determined exactly, but it may result from HIV infection of cells or inflammatory reactions to such infections.

■ aidsdrugs

an online database service of the National Library of Medicine with information about drugs undergoing testing against HIV infection, AIDS, AIDS-related complex and related opportunistic diseases.

■ AIDS Drug Assistance Program (ADAP)

a state program that provides drugs for HIV/AIDS and related opportunistic infections to individuals who otherwise could not afford them.

■ AIDS-related cancers

several cancers are more common or more aggressive in persons living with HIV. These malignancies include certain types of immune system cancers known as lymphomas, Kaposi's Sarcoma and anogenital cancers that primarily affect the anus and the cervix. HIV or the immune suppression it induces, appears to play a role in the development of these cancers.

■ AIDS Related Complex (ARC)

early Symptomatic HIV infection.

1. a group of common complications found in early stage HIV infection. They include progressive generalised lymphadenopathy (PGL), recurrent fever, unexplained weight loss, swollen lymph nodes, diarrhoea, herpes, hairy leukoplakia, fungus infection of the mouth and throat and/or the presence of HIV antibodies.
2. Symptoms that appear to be related to the infection by HIV. They include an unexplained, chronic deficiency of white blood cells (leukopenia) or a poorly functioning lymphatic sys-

tem with swelling of the lymph nodes (lymphadenopathy) lasting for more than three months without the opportunistic infections required for a diagnosis of AIDS.

AIDS-Related Dementia (ARD)

see AIDS dementia complex.

AIDS Service Organisation (ASO)

an organisation that provides care, education and/or other services to people with HIV/AIDS.

AIDS Vaccine Evaluation Group (AVEG)

a NIAID-sponsored network that conducts trials of experimental HIV vaccines at research centres called AIDS Vaccine Evaluation Units (AVEU).

AIDS Wasting Syndrome

the involuntary weight loss of 10 percent of baseline body weight plus either chronic diarrhoea (two loose stools per day for more than 30 days) or chronic weakness and documented fever (for 30 days or more, intermittent or constant) in the absence of a concurrent illness or condition other than HIV infection that would explain the findings.

AIN

see **Anal Intraepithelial Neoplasia.**

albumin

a protein found in bodily tissues and fluids, the principal protein in blood plasma. A reduced level of albumin in the serum of persons with AIDS-related wasting syndrome is a sign of progressive wasting and suggests a high risk of death.

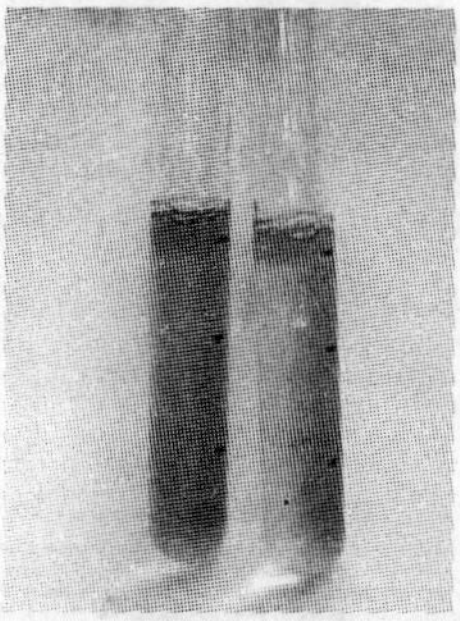

Alkaline Phosphatase (Alk Phos)

an enzyme. Doctors sometimes look for alkaline phosphatase to determine the condition of a patient's liver. Low counts are best. A high count suggests hepatitis or a drug toxicitity. (also abbreviated as alk phos).

alkaloid

a complex organic compound derived from plants, that contains nitrogen. Many alkaloids have pharmacological effects.

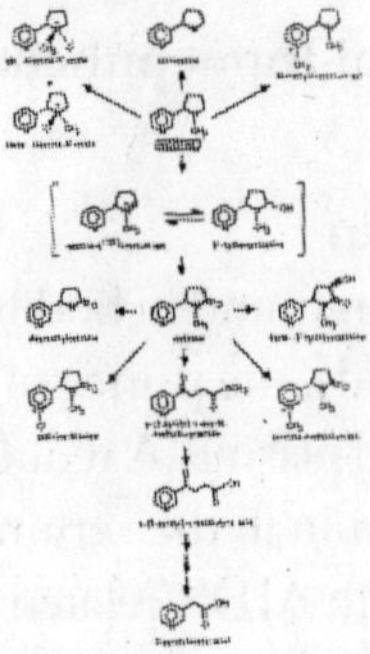

■ **allele**

a 'version' of a specific gene. Each individual has 1 allele at each specific genetic location.

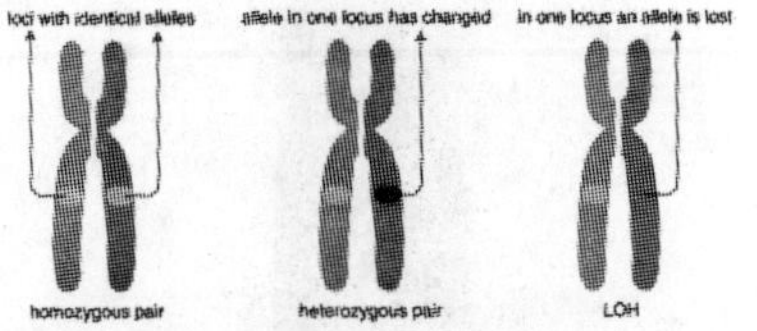

Schematic rendition of a pair of homologous chromosomes under conditions of homozygosity, heterozygosity and LOH. Homologous chromosomes are those pair during mitosis, have the same morphology, and contain genes governing the same characteristics. Note that one of the chromosomes, say the blue one, came from the father, and the other, the red, from the mother.

■ **allergen**

an agent or substance that stimulates an allergic or hypersensitivity reaction.

■ **allergy**

1. hypersensitivity to some environmental agent or drug. Most allergic reactions are minor (sneezing, runny nose), but some are life-threatening and require prompt medical attention.

2. n immune response to an antigen, i.e. allergen that does not normally cause an adverse reaction, e.g., animal dander, pollen. Allergic reactions are mediated by the release of histamine by mast cells. Allergic symptoms may include runny nose (rhinitis), sneezing, skin rash, asthma or anaphylactic shock.

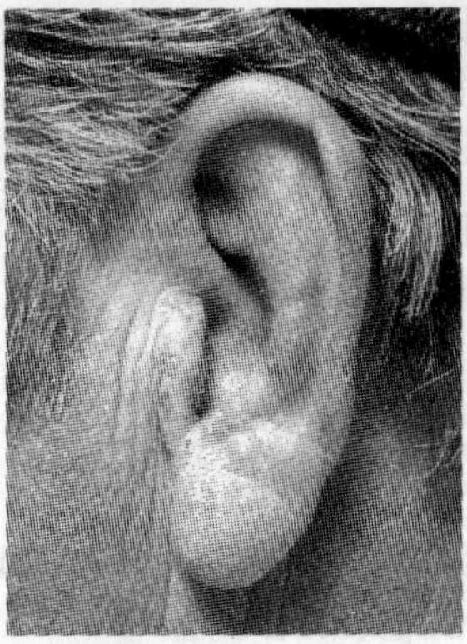

■ **allogenic**

refers to a graft or transfer, e.g. of tissue from a genetically non-identical individual.

■ **allograft**

a transplant from a genetically non-identical individual, i.e., someone other than an identical twin.

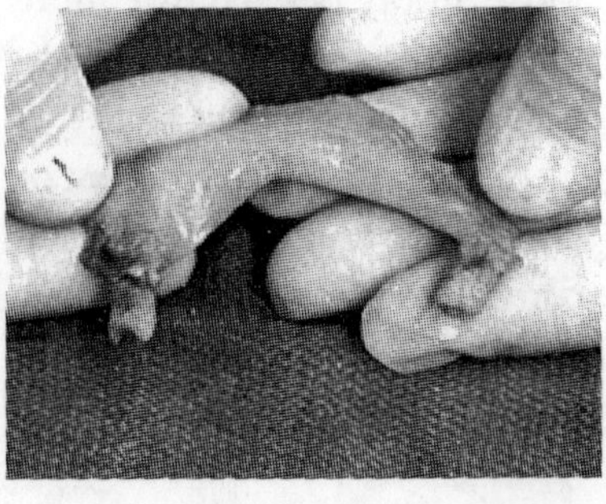

allopathy (adjective allopathic)
'Western medicine'. A therapeutic system in which illness or disease is treated by producing a second condition that is antagonistic towards or incompatible with the first, e.g., an antibiotic drug is given to treat infection with a micro-organism.

alopecia
hair loss.

alpha tocopherol
see **vitamin E.**

Alternative Therapy
therapy that is not considered standard practice in most Western countries, e.g., Traditional Chinese Medicine, homeopathy.

alum
an odourless, colourless substance used as a topical antibiotic, as an adjuvant in some vaccines and sometimes as placebo.

alveolus (plural alveoli)
the tiny sacs in the lung where oxygen and carbon dioxide are exchanged by red blood cells. Alveoli are the terminations of the bronchial tubes, where each sac is about .25 mm in size and there are approximately 1.5 million in each lung.

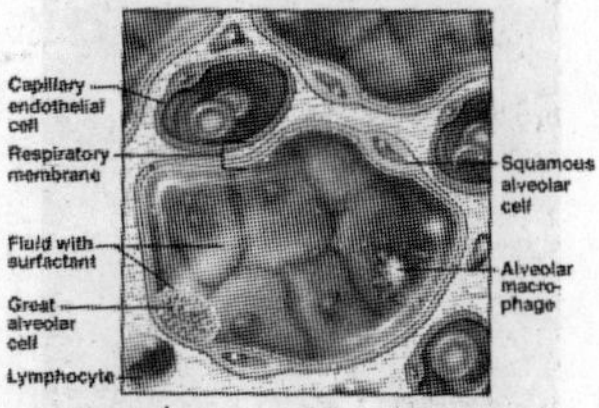

ambulatory
able to walk and move about without assistance. Ambulatory care typically refers to medical care received on an outpatient basis.

amoebiasis
infection with amoebas, a type of protozoan, especially Entamoeba histolytica. Amoebas invade the bowel mucosa causing ulceration and bloody diarrhoea. Transmission is by contaminated water or oral-facal transfer.

ameliorate
to make better or more tolerable.

amenorrhoea
absence of menstruation or decreased menstrual flow.

American Foundation For Aids Research (AMFAR)
a non-profit organisation that supports HIV/AIDS prevention and research efforts.

amino acid
one of 20+ organic acids that are the building blocks of proteins.

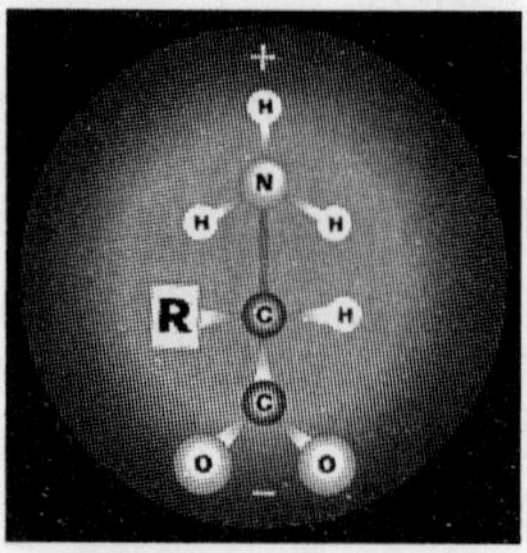

■ **aminoglycoside**

a family of antibiotic drugs similar to streptomycin.

■ **aminotransferase**

see **transaminase.**

■ **amniocentesis**

a procedure in which a needle is used to withdraw fluid from the amniotic sac that surrounds the foetus in the uterus for diagnosis, e.g. genetic analysis.

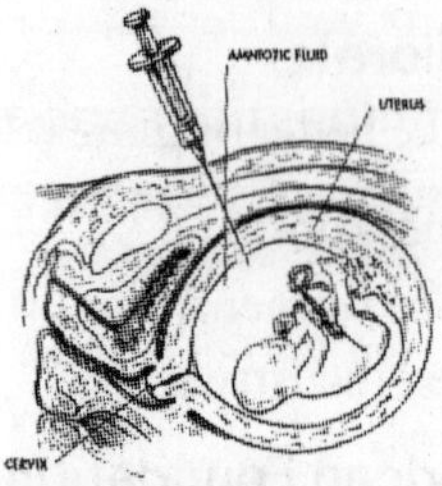

■ **amniotic fluid**

the fluid contained within the amnion or innermost membrane of the uterus, that envelopes the foetus during pregnancy.

■ **amphetamine**

a psycho-stimulant drug that acts on the central nervous system.

■ **Amphotericin B**

an antibiotic drug used to treat disseminated fungal infections, e.g. cryptococcal meningitis. The drug can have severe side effects including fever, chills, nausea, kidney toxicity and bone marrow suppression. Toxicity may be reduced by administering the drug in a liposomal, i.e. fat bubble form.

■ **amplification assay**

a type of test, e.g. polymerase chain reaction, branched-chain DNA, that detects small fragments of DNA or RNA and amplifies the fragments (target amplification) or the chemical signals they produce (signal amplification). Such assays are used to detect micro-organisms in the blood and tissues.

■ **ampule**

a small, sealed glass container used to hold a solution for injection.

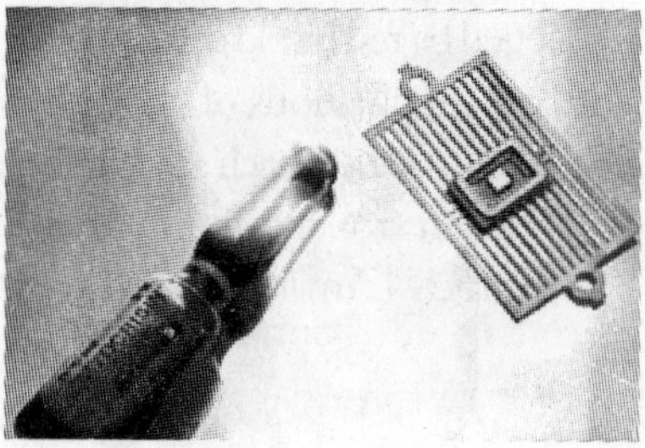

■ **amsler grid**

a diagram of squares used to assess vision. Defects in the central visual field, e.g. due to CMV retinitis, may be detected as breaks or unevenness in the lines of the grid.

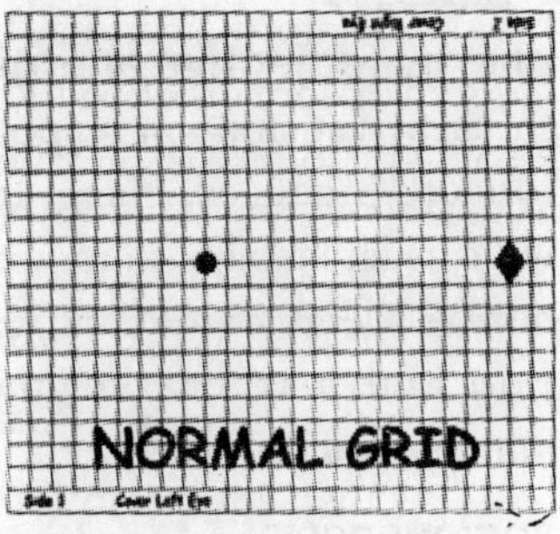

■ **amyl nitrite**

see **nitrite inhalant.**

■ **amylase**

an enzyme that converts starch to sugar. High levels in a lab test indicate pancreatitis as a possibility.

■ **anabolic steroid**

a synthetic hormone used to increase muscle size and strength.

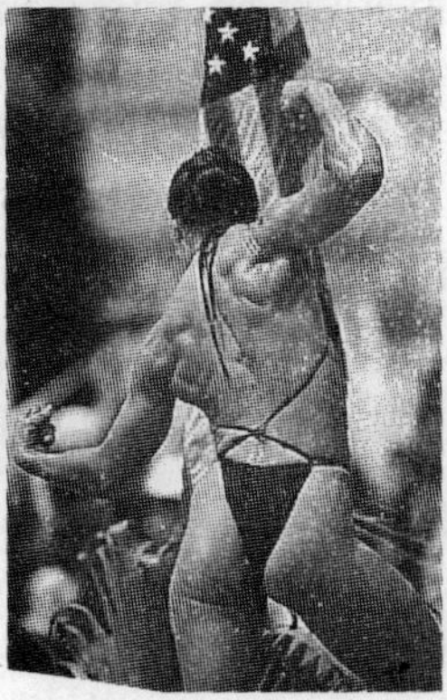

■ **anabolism**

the cellular synthesis of organic molecules. Amabolism is the building of proteins and muscle mass in the body.

■ **anaerobic**

living in the absence of oxygen e.g. anaerobic bacteria.

■ **Anal Intraepithelial Neoplasia (AIN)**

the abnormal growth of cells of the anus, which may be a precursor of anal cancer.

■ **analgesic**

a drug that reduces pain.

■ **analog**

variant of analogue.

■ **analogue**

a structural derivative.

■ **anamnestic response**

a heightened immunologic response stimulated by a second or subsequent exposure to a specific antigen.

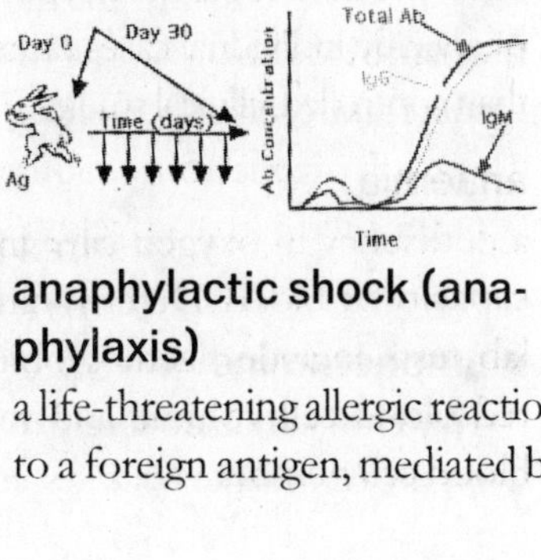

■ **anaphylactic shock (anaphylaxis)**

a life-threatening allergic reaction to a foreign antigen, mediated by

IgE antibodies. Symptoms include swelling, shortness of breath and a decrease in blood pressure due to capillary dilation.

■ **anatomy (adjective anatomic)**
the study of the structure of the body.

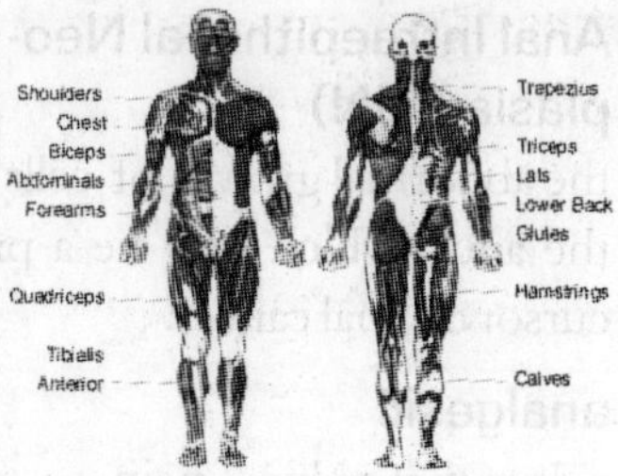

■ **androgen**
a hormone (e.g., testosterone androsterone) that has masculinising effects, including stimulation of the male reproductive organs and development of secondary sex characteristics. Androgens are produced by the testes and the adrenal glands.

■ **anecdotal**
refers to evidence based on reports of specific individual cases rather than controlled, clinical studies.

■ **anaemia**
a deficiency in oxygen-carrying capacity of blood. Determining lab tests include haemoglobin, red blood cell volume and red blood cell number.

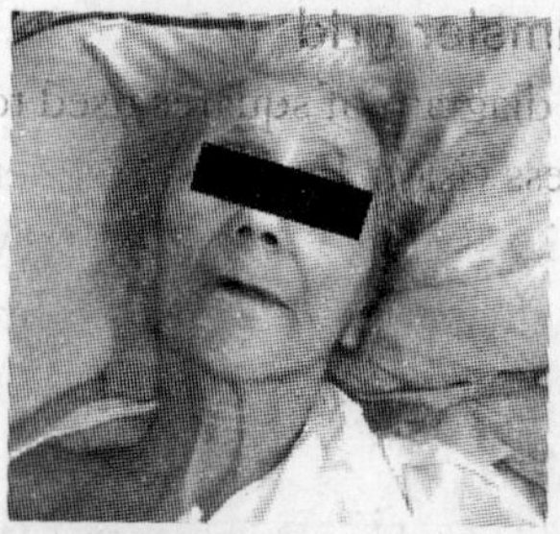

■ **anergy (adjective anergic)**
the lack of an immune response to a foreign antigen. Anergy may indicate an inability to mount a normal allergic or immune reaction and may be a sign of immunocompromise.

■ **angiogenesis**
the growth and proliferation of blood vessels.

■ **angiostatic**
an agent that inhibits the growth of new blood vessels.

■ **angular cheilitis**
see **cheilitis.**

■ **animal model**
a disease in an animal that resembles a similar disease in humans. Animal models are used to test new drugs and therapies.

■ **anogenital**
refers to the area that includes the genitals, perineum and anus.

■ **anorexia**
loss of appetite, especially as a result of disease.

■ **anoscopy**

examination of the anal canal and lower rectum using a short speculum.

■ **anova**

analysis of variance; a statistical technique that analyses the contribution to an experimental result made by independent variables.

■ **antagonist**

a drug that counteracts or neutralises another drug.

■ **antenatal**

the period of time before birth.

■ **anti-arrhythmic**

a drug that helps to normalize the rhythm of the heartbeat.

■ **anti-inflammatory**

acting against inflammation.

■ **antibacterial**

effective against bacteria, a substance that kills bacteria or halts bacterial replication.

■ **antibiotic**

an agent that inhibits the growth of or destroys micro-organisms. The term typically refers to an agent that is active against bacteria.

■ **antibody**

proteins in the blood that are generated in reaction to foreign proteins. Antibodies selectively neutralise the foreign proteins, producing immunity to certain microorganisms or their toxins. Tests to determine if you are HIV positive look for HIV antibodies, evidence that your body is attempting to fight the virus.

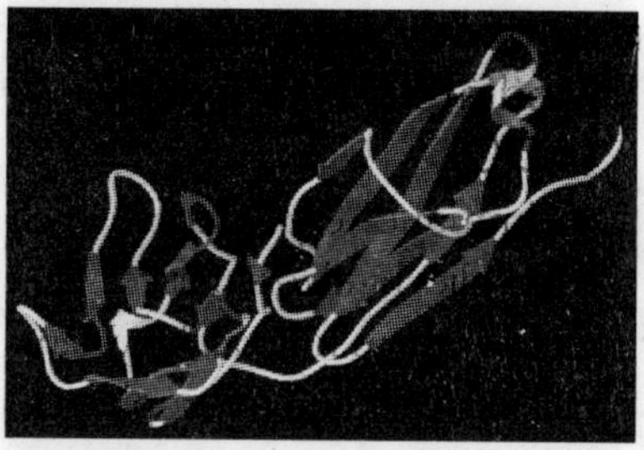

■ **antibody (ab, immunoglobulin, Ig)**

an immunoglobulin protein secreted by activated plasma cells, which evolve from B-cells. Antibodies are present throughout the blood and tissues. They are produced in response to stimulation by foreign antigens as part of the body's defence against disease. Specific antibodies bind to and act upon specific antigens. The antigen/antibody reaction forms the basis of humoral (TH2) immunity. Neutralising antibodies destroy or inactivate infectious agents, while enhancing antibodies promote infection. There are 5 classes of immunoglobulins: IgA, IgD, IgE, IgG and IgM.

antibody positive

having antibodies (e.g., against HIV) in the blood, indicating previous exposure to an organism. Typically the terms seropositive and HIV positive are used to mean antibody positive.

Antibody-Dependent Cell-Mediated Cytotoxicity (ADC)

an immune response in which antibodies bind to target cells and identify them for attack by natural killer cells and macrophages.

anticoagulant

a substance that suppresses blood clotting.

anticonvulsant

an agent that prevents or lessens convulsions or seizures; may be used as an adjuvant analgesic.

antidepressant

an agent that elevates the mood and prevents or alleviates psychological depression. Antidepressant drugs are sometimes used as adjuvant analgesic to relieve neuropathic pain. Heterocyclic and tricyclic classifications refer to antidepressants with specific chemical structures. Other classes of antidepressants include MAO inhibitors and serotonin reuptake inhibitors (e.g., Prozac).

antiemetic

an agent that relieves nausea and vomitting.

antifungal

a substance which kills fungus.

antigen

1. a substance that when introduced into the body stimulates production of an antibody.
2. any agent or substance that stimulates an immune response. Antigens are often foreign microorganisms such as bacteria or viruses or the substances they produce.

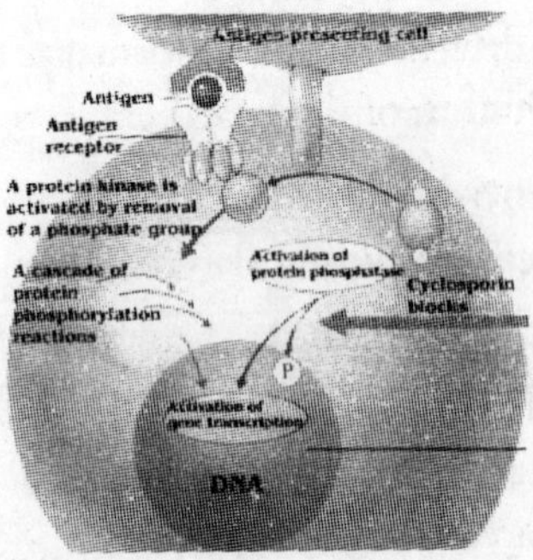

antigen positive

having proteins from a microorganism (e.g., HIV RNA) in the blood or tissues, as determined by tests such as the PCR assay.

Antigen-Presenting Cell (APC)

a cell, e.g., macrophage, that processes antigen proteins and displays the short peptide fragments on its surface in conjunction with Major Histocompatibility (MHC) proteins, enabling recognition by T-cells.

■ **antigenemia**
the presence of antigens in the blood.

■ **antihistamine**
an agent that counteracts the effects of histamine; antihistamines are used to treat allergic reactions and to block stomach acid production.

■ **antimicrobial**
an agent that destroys or prevents the growth of micro-organisms such as bacteria, fungi or parasites.

■ **antimycobacterial**
an agent that is active against mycobacteria (e.g., M. avium, M. tuberculosis).

■ **antineoplastic**
an agent that inhibits or prevents the proliferation of cancer cells and the growth of tumours.

■ **antioxidant**
a substance that inhibits oxidation. In your blood stream, free radicals damage cells by oxidising them. Beta-carotine, vitamin C and vitamin E are considered antioxidants.

■ **antiretroviral**
a substance that kills or suppresses a retrovirus, such as HIV. All of the anti-HIV drugs — AZT, protease inhibitors, etc. — are considered antiretroviral drugs.

■ **antisense**
the opposite (mirror image) of a genetic sequence, used to inactivate a genetic sequence.

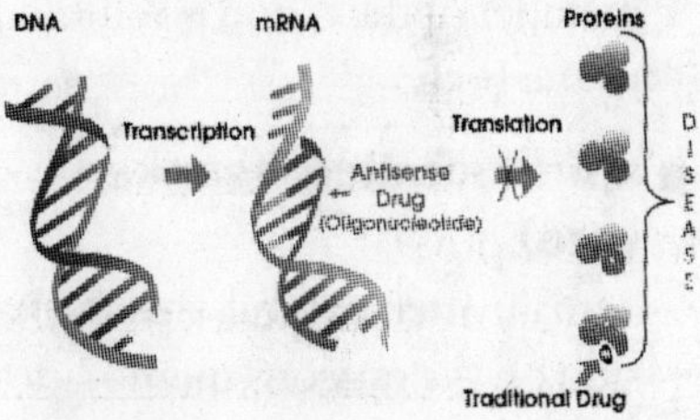

■ **antitoxin**
an antibody that recognises and neutralises a toxin, e.g. insect venom, bacterial toxins.

■ **antiviral**
a substance that kills or suppresses a virus.

■ **Antiviral Drug Advisory Committee**
a group of medical experts and advocates who make recommendations to the FDA regarding the approval of antiviral drugs.

■ **anxiolytic**
an agent, e.g. diazepam, that re-

duces the symptoms of anxiety.

■ aphasia
loss of the ability to speak or understand language.

■ apheresis
the removal of a specific component of the blood for therapeutic purposes, e.g. plasmapheresis or removal of plasma. Blood is removed, the desired components are filtered out and the remainder of the blood is returned to the body.

■ aphthous ulcer (canker sore)
a small, often painful, shallow lesion on the mucous membranes lining the mouth, oesophagus or rectum. Recurrent aphthous ulcers (RAU) reappear frequently and are refractory to treatment.

■ apoptosis
programmed cell death. Apoptosis is the body's mechanism for eliminating undesirable or excessive immune system activity, e.g. immune cells that attack the body's own tissues. Abnormal apoptosis is often seen in HIV disease.

■ arachidonic acid
an essential fatty acid that is a building block of prostaglandins and a component of cell membranes.

■ arc
abbreviation, AIDS Related Complex. A person with HIV who has symptoms but not severe enough to be classified as having AIDS.

■ arm
a group of participants in a research trial who receive the same treatment, i.e. treatment arm or placebo, i.e. control arm.

■ arrhythmia
loss of normal rhythm, especially irregularities of the heartbeat.

■ arthralgia
pain in a joint.

■ arthritis (plural arthritides)
inflammation of a joint, rheumatism.

■ artifact
an 'accidental' result or outcome that does to reflect reality, often due to an extraneous factor.

■ ascorbic acid (ascorbate)
see **vitamin C.**

■ ASO
see AIDS service organisation.

■ aspartate transaminase (ast, sgot)
see **transaminase.**

aspergilloma
a fungal mass that grows in a cavity in the lungs.

aspergillosis
a disease caused by a fungus. It can cause lesions of the skin, ear orbit, nasal sinuses, lungs and sometimes the bones, meninges, heart, kidneys or spleen. Symptoms include fever, chills, difficulty breathing and coughing up blood. If the infection reaches the brain, it may cause dementia.

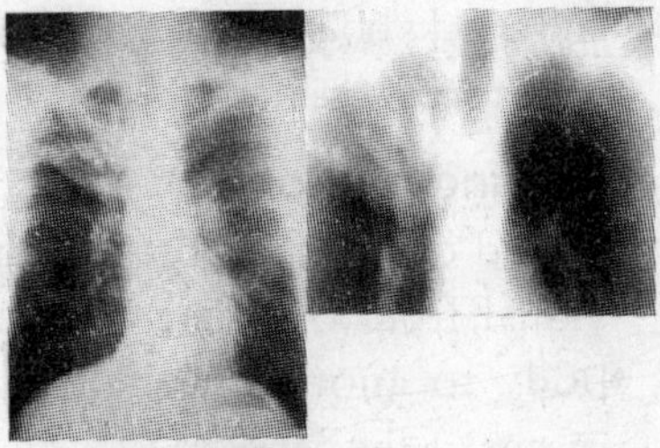

aspiration
withdrawal of fluid or tissue by suction, typically through a needle, e.g. to obtain a sample for analysis.

assay
qualitative (condition) or quantitative (amount) analysis of a substance, a test.

asthenia
weakness.

astrocyte
a cell within the brain that provides support for neurons and manufactures the myelin insulation that surrounds neuronal axons.

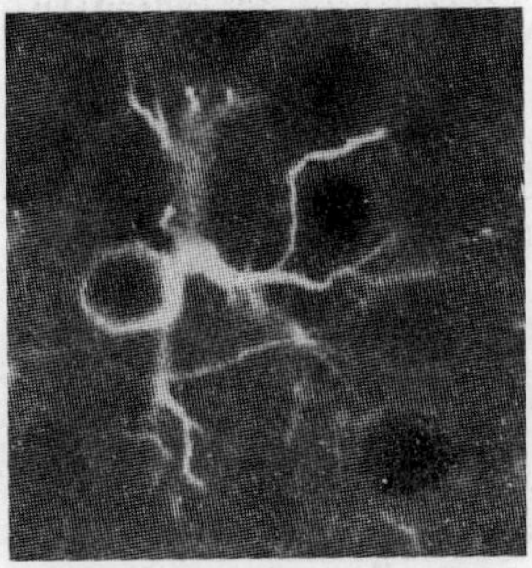

astrogliosis
proliferation of astrocytes within the brain.

asymptomatic
without symptoms, e.g. someone who is infected by HIV but has no symptoms.

ataxia
loss or lack of muscle coordination.

atevirdine
a non-nucleoside, reverse-transcriptase, antiretroviral drug.

atherosclerosis
'hardening of the arteries' in which cholesterol and other deposits build up on the inner walls of the artery, limiting the flow of blood.

athymic
lacking a thymus gland.

■ **atom**

the smallest division of an element that can exist independently. Atoms are made up of protons, neutrons and electrons and are the component parts of molecules.

■ **atovaquone (mepron, formerly 566c80)**

an anti-microbial drug used as a treatment for PCP, for individuals who cannot tolerate or fail on TMP-SMX and for pregnant women.

■ **atrophy**

1. emaciation, loss of tissue.
2. progressive degeneration, wasting or decrease in size, especially the loss of muscle tissue.

■ **attenuate**

to weaken or reduce the level of virulence. An attenuated virus has a diminished ability to cause disease and may be used in vaccines.

■ **atypia**

a condition of being abnormal or not typical.

■ **auto-antibodies**

an antibody thought to act against cells of the organism in which it is formed.

■ **autocrine**

a cellular messenger that acts at or near the site where it is produced.

■ **autoimmune**

related to or caused by auto-antibodies. A disease where the body's cells attacks themselves.

■ **autoimmune response (autoimmunity)**

a condition, e.g. rheumatoid arthritis, systemic lupus erythematosus in which an individual's immune system fails to recognize its own biochemical markers as being 'self' and attacks bodily tissues as if they were foreign matter.

■ **autoinoculation**

spread of infection by an individual from one part of their body to another, usually by means of the hands.

■ **autologous**

derived from the same individual. An autologous transfusion or transplant is one in which a person's own blood or tissues are removed and reintroduced at a later time.

■ **Autonomic Nervous System (ANS)**

the branch of the nervous system that primarily controls nonvoluntary bodily processes such as heartbeat, intestinal motility and non-endocrine gland secretion.

The ANS has two branches, sympathetic and parasympathetic.

■ **autopsy (post mortem)**
a physical examination and/or dissection of a body following death.

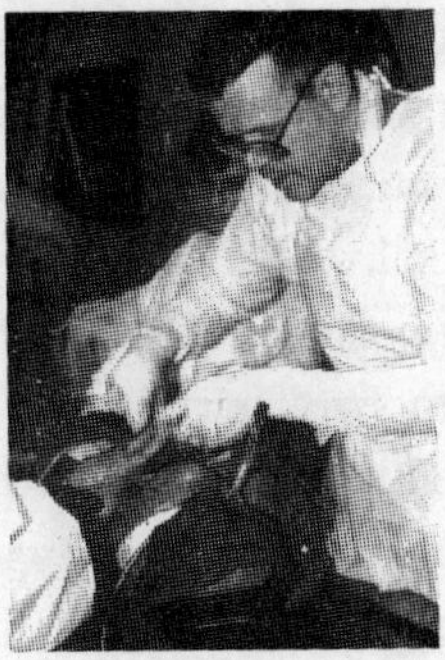

■ **aviremia**
lack of virus in the blood plasma.

■ **axon**
the long structure of a nerve cell that acts as a pathway for nerve impulses.

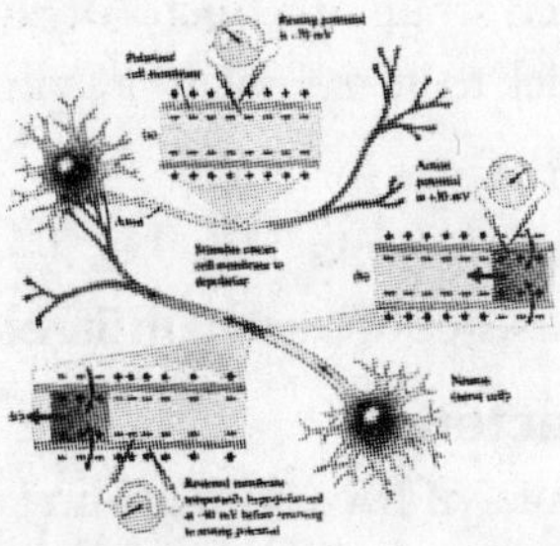

■ **ayurvedic**
a system of traditional medicine practiced in India.

■ **azidothymidine**
see **AZT.**

■ **azithromycin (zithromax)**
a macrolide antibiotic used to treat Mycobacterium avium complex (MAC) disease, chlamydiasis and urinary tract infections.

■ **azole drug**
a class of drugs used to fight fungal infections. There are 2 subclasses, the imidazoles (e.g., clotrimazole, ketoconazole) and the triazoles (e.g., fluconazole, itraconazole).

■ **AZT**
a nucleoside (thymidine) analog drug that suppresses the replication of HIV by terminating DNA synthesis. AZT is FDA-approved for the treatment of HIV infection; current practice favours the use of AZT in combination with other antiretroviral drugs. AZT crosses the blood-brain barrier and may be effective against AIDS dementia complex. Adverse side effects include nausea, myopathy and bone marrow suppression.

■ **aztec**
a controlled-release formulation of AZT.

■ **b complex**
see **vitamin B.**

■ b-cell (b-lymphocyte)
an immune system white blood cell that carries out the humoral (TH2) immune response. B-cells are produced in the bone marrow and mature into plasma cells that produce antibodies. B-cells are influenced by various cytokines and interactions with T-cells and other immune system components.

■ b-cells
common term for B-lymphocyte cells.

■ b-lymphocytes
also called B-cells — blood cells derived from bone marrow and the spleen. They are able to detect foreign objects and produce antibodies. B-cells are activated by T-lymphocytes.

■ b.i.d.
pharmaceutical abbreviation, two times a day (*bis in die*).

■ b.i.w.
pharmaceutical abbreviation, two times a week.

■ bacille calmette-guérin
an attenuated strain of Mycobacterium bovis. BCG is used in some countries as a vaccine against tuberculosis. BCG vaccination renders the PPD test unusable as a test for the presence of M. tuberculosis. BCG adenitis is an illness caused by BCG that is present in some infants with HIV and is characterised by inflammation of the lymph nodes.

■ bacilliary angiomatosis (cat scratch disease)
a vascular proliferative disease caused by Bartonella henselae or Bartonella quintana that may result in swollen purplish lesions similar to those of Kaposi's sarcoma. BA is associated with contact with domestic cats.

■ bacillus (plural bacilli)
a type of gram-positive, rod-shaped bacteria typically found in soil.

■ back-mutation
the reversion of a mutant, attenuated strain of a micro-organism back to its natural, more virulent state.

■ bacteremia
presence of bacteria in the blood.

■ bacteria
plural of bacterium, are tiny, one-cell organisms of the class Schizomycetes. There is a vast assortment of bacteria, including many parasites.

■ Bacterial Vaginosis (BV)
a condition caused by the overgrowth of anaerobic bacteria, e.g. Gardnerella vaginalis, resulting in vaginal irritation and discharge.

■ bactericide
an agent that kills or neutralises bacteria.

■ bacteriostatic
an agent that inhibits bacterial growth or reproduction but does not kill bacteria. Contrast with bactericide.

■ bacterium (plural bacteria)
a simple single-celled micro-organism, are classified by their shape (rod, spirochete), staining properties (Gram positive or Gram negative) and habitat (aerobic, anaerobic). Many types of bacteria are pathogenic in humans.

■ bactrim
a brand name of trimethoprim-sulfamethoxazole (TMP-SMX).

■ baculovirus
a virus of insects used in the production of some HIV vaccines.

■ balanitis
inflammation of the glans i.e. the head of the penis.

■ band
an immature neutrophil released into the bloodstream to combat infection.

■ barbiturate
a class of drugs, e.g. phenobarbital that have sedative properties and depress respiratory rate, blood pressure and nervous system activity.

■ bartonella
a species of bacteria associated with diseases including bacterial angiomatosis (cat-scratch disease), trench fever and endocarditis (heart infection).

■ basal
refers to the base or lowest level.

■ basal cell
a skin cell located in one of the innermost layers of the skin.

■ Basal Cell Epithelioma (BCE)
basal cell skin cancer which appears as a pink raised patch with a necrosed centre. A left untreated, the lesion may invade deeper tissues. In otherwise healthy people, BCE tends to occur on areas of the body exposed to the sun, but in HIV-infected people, it may occur on unexposed areas.

■ basal ganglion (plural ganglia)
a cluster of nerve tissue, primarily composed of neuron cell bodies, deep within the brain.

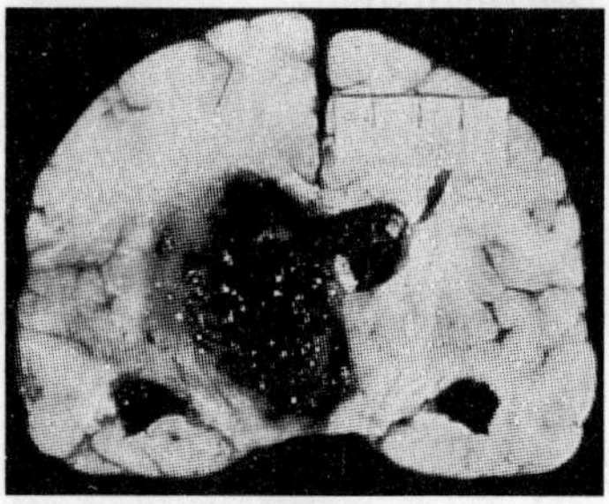

■ Basal Metabolic Rate(BMR)
the body's resting level of energy expenditure. Individuals with a chronic infection often have an elevated basal metabolic rate.

■ base line
a line used as a base for measurement. In HIV Disease, a base line is the results of several lab tests used to monitor the effectiveness of drugs. (Commonly — but incorrectly — spelled as a single word: baseline).

■ base-pairing
the process by which a nucleic acid base matches up with its complementary counterpart during replication of genetic material, e.g. Adenine (A) pairs with Thymine (T) or Uracil (U). Cytosine (C) pairs with Guanine (G).

■ baseline
an initial or known value, e.g. CD4 cell count, HIV viral load to which later measurements can be compared.

■ Basic Fibroblast Growth Factor (BFGF)
a cytokine that promotes blood vessel proliferation, which is essential for the development of Kaposi's sarcoma and other neoplasms.

■ basophil
a type of white blood cell (granulocyte) that releases chemicals in allergic reactions. Basophils that leave the bloodstream become mast cells in the tissues.

■ BCG
see **bacille calmette-guerin.**

■ BDNA
abbreviation for branched DNA assay See branched DNA assay.

■ Beck Depression Index
a written self-report questionnaire used to measure clinical depression.

■ benign
refers to a mild, non-lethal illness, especially a non-cancerous neoplasm. Contrast with malignant.

■ **beta carotene**
a reddish-orange antioxidant pigment found in dark yellow or orange fruits and vegetables. Beta carotene is a precursor of Vitamin A that is stored in the liver and converted as needed.

■ **beta interferon**
see **interferon.**

■ **Beta-2 Microglobulin (B2M)**
a cell surface protein that is released into the bloodstream when cells die. Elevated blood levels of B2M are associated with immune activation and HIV replication. Levels below 3 mg/litre are considered normal; levels above 5 mg/litre indicate a high risk of HIV disease progression.

■ **BHAP**
bisheteroarlypiperazine, a class of non-nucleoside reverse transcriptase inhibitor antiviral drugs (e.g., atevirdine, delavirdine).

■ **BHCG**
see **human chorionic gonadotropin.**

■ **bias**
a false association that results from the failure to account for some skewing or influencing factor or a tendency for the observed results to deviate from the 'true' results. Bias distorts results in a particular direction. For example, if an investigator in a clinical trial believes the drug under study to be effective and knows which participants are receiving the drug, bias may influence his/her observations in favour of positive results.

■ **biaxin**
brand name of clarithromycin.

■ **bid**
pharmaceutical abbreviation, twice a day.

■ **bilateral**
occurring on both sides, e.g. of the body.

■ **biliary system**
a digestive subsystem that is important for the digestion of fats. Bile is produced by the liver and stored in the gallbladder until needed.

■ **bilirubin**
a reddish-yellow compound that occurs naturally in bile, blood and urine.. Too much bilirubin indicates there may be a liver problem.

■ **bioavailability**
the degree a drug or nutrient is available to the body. Bioavailability is influenced by

how much the substance is absorbed and circulated.

■ Bioelectrical Impedence Analysis (BIA)
a method of measuring lean body mass (muscle) and estimating cell mass. BIA measures electrical resistance and capacitative reactance and uses these values to calculate phase angle.

■ bioflavonoid (vitamin p)
an antioxidant substance, e.g. rutin, esculin derived from plants that has a variety of biological activities.

■ biohazard
a danger to humans, animals or the environment caused by a biological agent or condition.

■ Biological Response Modifier (BRM)
an immuno-modulator; an agent, e.g. cytokine, thymic hormone that enhances or restores immune function.

■ biomicroscopy
see **colposcopy.**

■ biopsy
the study of tissue taken from a living body or organism, especially in the search for disease. A biopsy is often as simple as cutting off a small amount of skin, but other cases are more invasive.

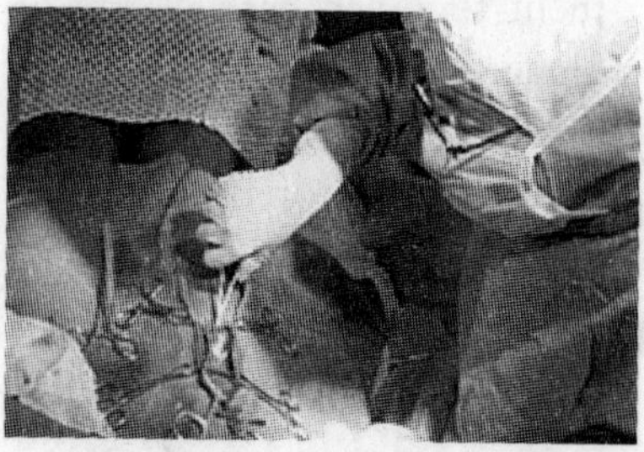

■ biotechnology
industrial processes that involve the use of biological systems or their products, e.g. monoclonal antibodies, recombinant proteins produced by genetically engineered bacteria.

■ birg587
see **nevirapine.**

■ bitter melon (momordica charantia)
a plant with a long tradition of medicinal use in Asia. The plant is a source of MAP 30, a protein that shows anti-HIV activity in vitro.

■ blastogenesis
the production and maturation of new lymphocytes in response to challenge by an infectious agent, e.g. bacterium, virus.

■ blastomycosis
an infectious disease caused by a fungus, usually in the lungs. It can

spread to the skin, bone or other tissues.

■ blinding
a method of conducting clinical trials so that some or all of the participants do not know whether subjects are taking active drug or placebo. Blinding is done to reduce bias in drug trials. See also double-blind.

■ blood chemistry panel
a set of tests, e.g. SMA 12, SMA 14, SMA 20 that evaluate the level of chemical components, e.g. glucose, albumin, enzymes, electrolytes in the blood.

■ blood transfusion
the infusion of blood or blood components into an individual for the treatment of a medical condition, e.g. anaemia, loss of blood due to injury. Transfused blood may be homologous (from a donor) or autologous (previously stored blood from the recipient).

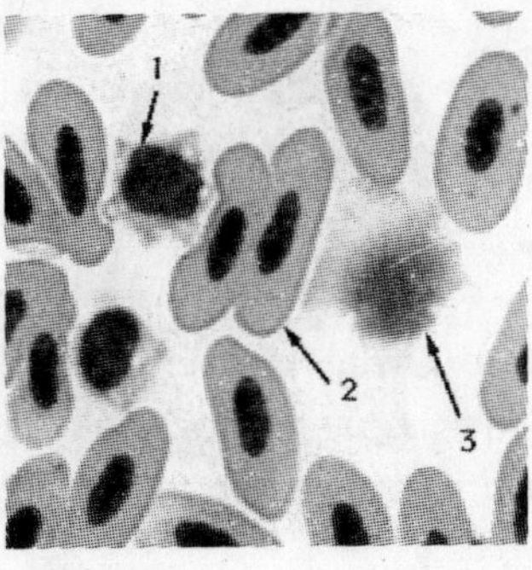

■ blood volume
the amount of blood circulating throughout the body in the vascular system. Normal adult blood volume is about 5 litres. Blood volume must be maintained to ensure the proper functioning of the heart, kidneys and other organs.

■ blood-brain barrier
a membrane separating brain tissue from circulating blood. In HIV treatment, it usually refers to the difficulty of getting drugs from the blood stream to penetrate into the central nervous system. HIV is active in brain tissue. The drug AZT crosses the blood-brain barrier better than any other anti-HIV drug.

■ bloodwork
laboratory tests that measure properties of the blood.

■ body cell mass
muscle and organ tissue.

■ body fluids
a group of fluids made within the body, usually blood, saliva, semen and urine.

■ Body Mass Index (BMI)
a measure of mass that is calculated as weight divided by height squar

■ **bone marrow**

see **marrow.**

■ **Bone Marrow Transfer (BMT)**

a graft of bone marrow from one individual to another to reconstitute the recipient's damaged immune system.

■ **booster**

a subsequent dose given some time after the initial administration of a vaccine or drug to enhance or restore its effectiveness.

■ **botanical**

a medicine or therapy prepared from plants or a herbal medicine.

■ **botulism**

life-threatening food poisoning caused by the presence of botulinus toxin produced by Clostridium botulinum bacteria. Cases in humans are usually associated with raw or improperly preserved foods, especially cured meats. Symptoms include nausea, vomitting, cramps, diarrhoea, vomitting, fatigue, dizziness, vision problems and headache. Severe cases may progress to symmetrical paralysis.

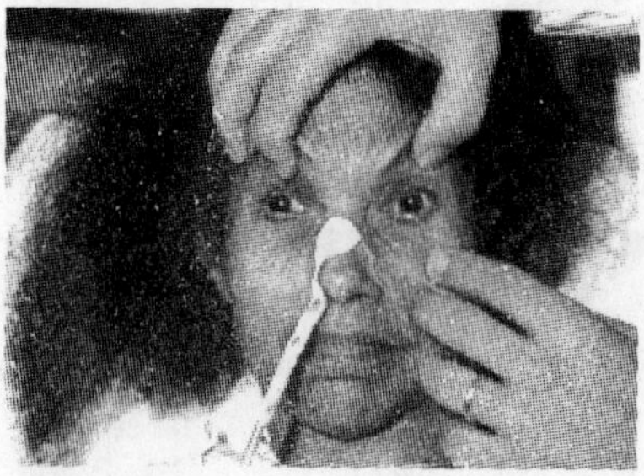

■ **bovine**

refers to cattle or that which is derived from cattle.

■ **bovine hyperimmune colostrum**

a compound derived from the colostrum (early breast secretions) of cows. Colostrum contains high levels of immunoglobulins.

■ **bowenoid papulosis**

a dysplastic disorder involving tissue changes in the anogenital region, including reddish raised or flat lesions. Bowenoid papulosis is associated with human papillomavirus, especially HPV type 16. If left untreated, it may progress to squamous cell carcinoma.

■ **brain stem**

the lower part of the brain where the brain connects to the spinal

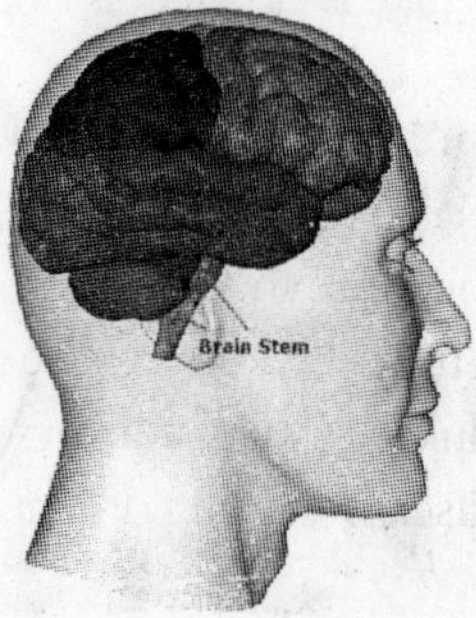

cord. The brain stem is responsible for many motor and sensory functions, especially automatic functions such as maintenance of posture.

■ **branched DNA assay**
a kind of test indicating the amount of HIV (or viral load) in the blood, commonly abbreviated bDNA.

■ **branched-chain DNA assay (bdna, quantiplex hiv rna)**
a test that measures the amount of virus (viral load) in plasma or tissue using a chemical signal, visible as light, that is produced by viral RNA.

■ **breakthrough**
refers to a condition that has developed despite measures to prevent it, e.g. PCP that occurs while taking a prophylactic drug.

■ **broad-spectrum antibiotic**
an antibiotic drug that is active against a range of different bacteria.

■ **bronchial lavage (bronchoalveolar lavage)**
a procedure in which the bronchial tubes are rinsed. The resulting fluid can then be analysed, e.g. for disease-causing organisms.

■ **bronchiole**
a small branch of the bronchial tubes or airway.

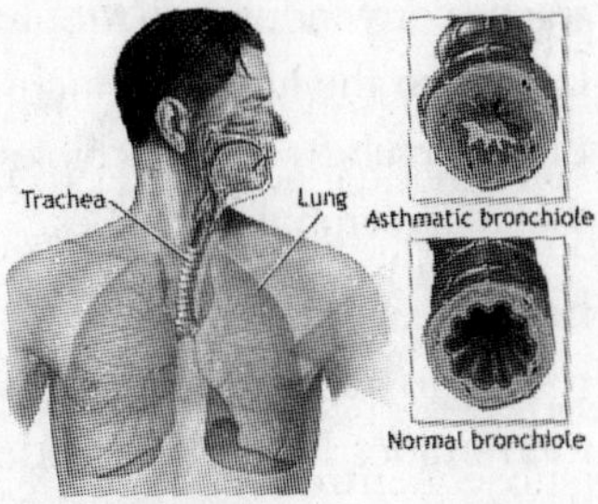

■ **bronchitis**
acute or chronic inflammation of the branched part of the trachea — the tubes going into the left and right lungs. In some cases, this is considered an AIDS-defining condition in the United States.

■ **bronchodilation**
opening or expanding the bronchial tubes. Bronchodilating drugs can reduce coughing, wheezing and/or shortness of breath and may help prevent coughing if given prior to therapy with aerosolised pentamidine.

■ **bronchoscopy**
procedure for examining the respiratory tract using a thin, flexible tube through the mouth and into the lungs.

■ **bronchospasm**
an involuntary contraction of the bronchial tubes, which may lead to breath difficulty.

bronchus (plural bronchi; adjective bronchial)
the airway tubes that lead from the trachea or windpipe to the alveolar sacs in the lungs. Bronchi are the larger tubes and bronchioles are the smallest tubule branches.

buccal
relating to the cheek, especially the membranes lining the inside of the cheek.

buffer
something that lessens or absorbs an impact. A buffered drug is commonly a tablet that has been coated with a substance that prevents stomach upset.

bulimia
an eating disorder characterised by binge eating followed by forced purging, by means of self-induced vomitting or use of laxatives.

burkitt's lymphoma
a cancer of the lymph system that is associated with the Epstein-Barr virus.

buyers' club
a non-profit organisation that sells drugs, vitamins, nutritional supplements and other therapies for HIV/AIDS. Many buyers' clubs sell drugs that are not approved and therefore not available in pharmacies.

bv-ara-u
see **sorivudine.**

cachexia
general wasting due to illness or stress.

caf
abbreviation, see **cell antiviral factor.**

calcium
a metallic trace element essential for bone maintenance and proper neural and muscular function. Calcium is found in dairy products and leafy green vegetables.

calorie
a unit of measurement of heat or energy.

campylobacter
a family of bacteria, e.g. C. jejuni, C. fetus, that may cause acute illness affecting the small intestine, characterised by abdominal pain, nausea, vomitting, fever and bloody diarrhoea. Campylobacter is frequently found in undercooked poultry and in raw or unpasteurised milk products.

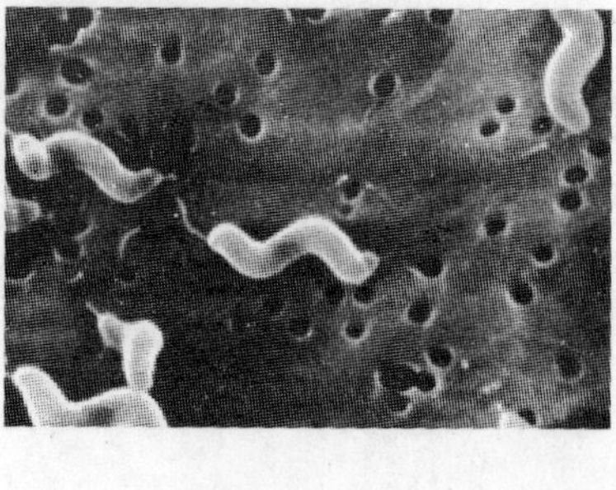

■ **canarypox**

a poxvirus that typically infects canaries and is used in human vaccine research.

■ **cancer**

a group of diseases characterised by abnormal growth (neoplasm, tumour) and spread to other parts of the body (metastasism).

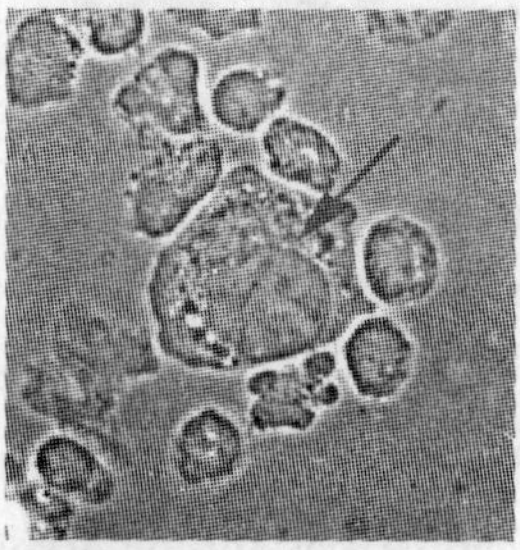

■ **candida**

a genus of yeast-like fungi. Some species of Candida are part of the normal flora of the mouth, intestines and vagina. Several species may cause infection in humans, especially immuno-compromised persons, including C. albicans, C. tropicalis and C. krusei.

■ **candidemia**

the presence of Candida in the peripheral blood.

■ **candidiasis**

a fungus infection, caused by a member of the genus Candida. In the mouth, candidiasis is called thrush and shows up as white patches. In the vagina, the disease is called vulvovaginal candidiasis. Candidiasis can also attack lungs and the oesophagus. This infection is considered as an AIDS-defining condition.

■ **canker sore**

see **aphthous ulcer.**

■ **cannabis**

cannabis sativa, a plant that contains the psychoactive ingredient delta-9 tetrahydrocannabinol (THC). Cannabis ingestion typically produces feelings of euphoria and/or drowsiness. Cannabis is used medically to reduce nausea due to chemotherapy and restore appetite in persons with wasting syndrome, commonly known as marijuana.

■ **capillaries**

tiny blood vessels that form the most distal part of the circulatory system. Arteries branch into even smaller vessels, finally ending in the capillaries, which connect with the smallest branches of the veins. Capillaries deliver oxygen and nutrients to and remove waste products from the body's cells.

■ **carbohydrate**

an organic molecule composed mainly of carbon, hydrogen and oxygen atoms. Carbohydrates constitute a major class of nutrients and are present in foods such as bread and pasta.

■ **carbon dioxide**

a colourless, odourless gas. Carbon dioxide is a by-product of cellular metabolism that is eliminated by the lungs. Carbon dioxide levels in the blood determine the breathing rate and the blood's acid-base balance.

■ **carcinogenesis**

the development of cancer. A carcinogen is a chemical or physical agent (e.g., drugs, radiation) that facilitates the development of cancer. (*adjective* carcinogenic).

■ **carcinoma**

a malignant tumour of the epithelial cells that line body surfaces and cavities. Carcinoma in situ (CIS) refers to an early stage of cancer that has not invaded surrounding tissues.

■ **cardiomyopathy**

a degeneration of the heart muscle, thought to be caused by HIV or by some drugs.

■ **cardiovascular**

refers to the circulatory system (the heart and blood vessels).

■ **carpal tunnel syndrome**

a condition in which a nerve in the wrist becomes inflamed and presses against the bones that make up the carpal tunnel, often resulting in pain. Carpal tunnel syndrome is often caused by repetitive strain and may also be a side effect of treatment with human growth hormone.

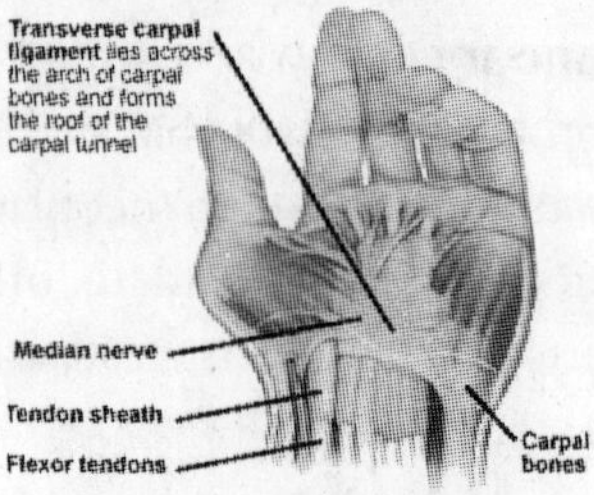

■ **castleman's disease**

a disease that causes benign enlargement (hyperplasia) of the lymph nodes.

■ **CAT scan**

also known as computed axial tomography, a medical technology that uses X rays and computers to produce three-dimensional images of the human body. It provides detailed views of the body's soft tissues, including blood vessels, muscle tissue and organs, such as the brain. The images produced by CAT scan depict a cross-section of the body.

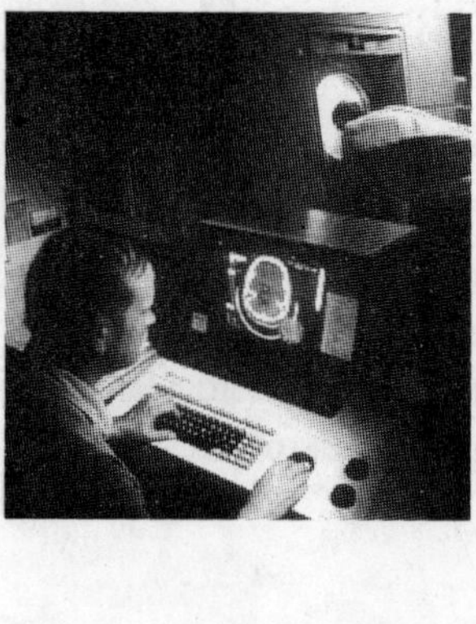

■ cat scratch disease
see **bacillary angiomatosis.**

■ catabolism
the breakdown of bodily proteins for energy and raw materials. Excess catabolism results in wasting.

■ catalyst
an agent that promotes or accelerates a chemical reaction without itself being consumed.

■ Category A, B, C (AIDS)
a system for classifying stages of HIV/AIDS. Category A indicates full-blown AIDS. Category B indicates illnesses and symptoms, e.g. Kaposi's sarcoma that qualify as an AIDS diagnosis. Category C indicates illnesses and symptoms, e.g. cervical intraepithelial neoplasia, that are attributable to or complicated by HIV infection, but which are not AIDS-defining.

■ Category A, b, D, D, X (DRUGS)
the FDA pregnancy risk categories that indicate risk to a foetus from maternal use of a drug. Category A drugs have not shown a risk in controlled studies. Category B drugs either have not been tested in animals or show adverse effects in animals which have not been confirmed in humans. Category C means that no controlled studies have been done in humans. Category D indicates that there is evidence of human foetal risk, but the benefits of the drug may outweigh the risk. Category X includes drugs which in animal and human studies (or common experience) have been shown to cause foetal abnormalities.

■ catheter
a flexible tube inserted into a body channel to maintain an opening to the channel. Catheters are commonly used in veins for ongoing drug treatment.

■ cautery
burning or cutting tissue by means of heat, chemicals or an electric current.

■ cavitating
creating holes. Used to describe the effect active tuberculosis has on lung tissue.

■ CBC
abbreviation, Complete Blood Count. A battery of blood tests, including counts of various cells, hematocrig and haemoglobin.

■ CC
abbreviation, Cubic centimetre, often used as a unit of measurement for drug dosages.

■ **CCR5**
abbreviation, see **CKR5.**

■ **CD4**
a protein embedded in the surface of some T-cells and certain other cells (e.g., macrophages, Langerhans cells, glial cells). HIV invades cells by attaching to their CD4 receptor.

■ **CD4 count**
the number of helpter T-lymphocytes in a patients blood, usually expressed as the number of cells per cubic millimetre. When this value drops below 200, the patient has AIDS. Also called T cell count.

■ **CD4/CD8 ratio**
the ratio of CD4 cells to CD8 cells. In healthy individuals the CD4/CD8 ratio is about 2.

■ **CD8 (t8)**
protein embedded in the surface of killer and suppressor T-lymphocytes. Blood tests that look for suppressor T-lymphocytes are actually looking for this protein.

■ **CDC**
abbreviation, Centres for Disease Control and Prevention — an agency of the U.S. Department of Health and Human Services, located in Atlanta, Georgia. CDC is on mission to promote health and quality of life by preventing and controlling disease, injury and disability.

■ **ceiling effect**
the phenomenon in which a drug reaches a maximum effect, so that increasing the drug dosage does not increase its effectiveness.

■ **cell**
the smallest structural unit of an organism that is capable of independent functioning. A cell consists of a nucleus, cytoplasm, various organelles and inanimate matter, all surrounded by a semipermeable plasma membrane.

■ **Cell Antiviral Factor (CAF)**
a factor produced by CD8 cells that is hypothesised to block viral infection during the HIV latency period and in long-term non-progressors. The identity of this factor is not known; possibilities include IL-16 and the chemokines RANTES, MIP-1-alpha and MIP-1-beta.

■ **cell cycle**
the sequence of events that a cell goes through in the process of replication. The cycle consists of 4 stages: G1, a resting stage prior to replication; S, in which DNA is synthesised; G2, a 'gap' stage;

and M, in which mitotic cell division takes place.

■ **cell expansion**
an immuno-modulating therapy in which cytotoxic T-lymphocytes are removed from the body of an HIV-infected person, treated with IL-2 to induce proliferation and re-infused into the person in order to strengthen the cell-mediated immune response.

■ **cell line**
a specific type of cell that is maintained in vitro for medical and/or research purposes.

■ **cell membrane**
the envelope around a cell which encloses the cytoplasm and is responsible for the exchange of materials with the surrounding environment.

■ **cell-associated virus**
virus that resides within a host cell. Contrast with cell-free virus.

■ **cell-free virus**
virus that exists outside of cells within the bloodstream. Contrast with cell-associated virus.

■ **cell-mediated immunity**
part of the immune system responsible for directly attacking foreign material without using proteins (antibodies), consists mainly of T-lymphocytes, killer cells and macrophages.

■ **cellulitis**
an inflammation of subcutaneous connective tissue.

■ **Centres For Disease Control And Prevention (CDC)**
the U.S. federal government agency within the Public Health Service of the Department of Health and Human Services that monitors disease occurrence and develops policies for preventing diseases and maintaining the health of the population.

■ **centi-**
prefix, one-hundredth.

■ **cento-**
prefix, one hundred times.

■ **central nervous system**
a network in the body consisting of the brain, spinal cord and nerves, commonly abbreviated CNS.

■ **cephalosporin**
a class of antibiotic drugs similar to penicillin.

■ **cerebellum**
the lower back part of the brain responsible for functions such as maintaining balance and coordinating and controlling voluntary muscle movement.

cerebrospinal
relating to the brain and spinal cord.

Cerebrospinal Fluid (CSF)
a clear, nutrient-rich fluid that circulates around and through the brain and around the spinal cord.

cerebrum
the upper frontal part of the brain responsible for thought and for higher motor functions and sensory processing. The term cerebral is often used to refer to the brain in general.

cervical cancer
in women only. Malignant growth in the narrow lower or outer end of the uterus, in some cases, this is considered an AIDS-defining condition.

cervical dysplasia
in women only. Abnormal tissue growth in the narrow lower or outer end of the uterus, this can lead to cervical cancer.

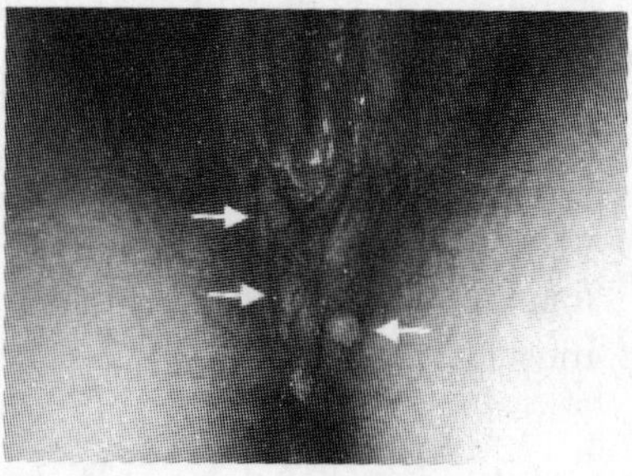

Cervical Intraepithelial Neoplasia (CIN)
abnormal growth of cells of the uterine cervix, suggesting an early stage of cervical cancer. Human papillomavirus (HPV) and HIV infection are associated with an increased risk of CIN. There are 3 grades of severity: CIN I, CIN II and CIN III. A newer classification system divides these 3 classes into 2 categories: low-grade and high-grade squamous intraepithelial lesion (SIL).

cervicitis
inflammation of the uterine cervix.

cervix
the cylindrical, lower part of the uterus leading into the vagina. (*adjective* cervical).

caesarean section
a delivery procedure that involves making an incision through the abdominal wall to remove an infant from the uterus.

CFIDS
abbreviation, Chronic Fatigue Immune Dysfunction Syndrome. See **Chronic Fatigue Syndrome.**

CFS
abbreviation, see **Chronic Fatigue Syndrome.**

chancre

a red, painless ulcer. A primary sore or lesion that forms at the site of entry of a micro-organism, e.g. the spirochete bacterium that causes syphilis.

chancroid

a sexually transmitted disease caused by infection with Haemophilus ducreyi, it is characterised by soft chancres or ulcers.

cheilitis

inflammation and fissures radiating from the corners of the mouth. Cheilitis may be due to various causes, e.g., nutritional deficiencies, candidiasis.

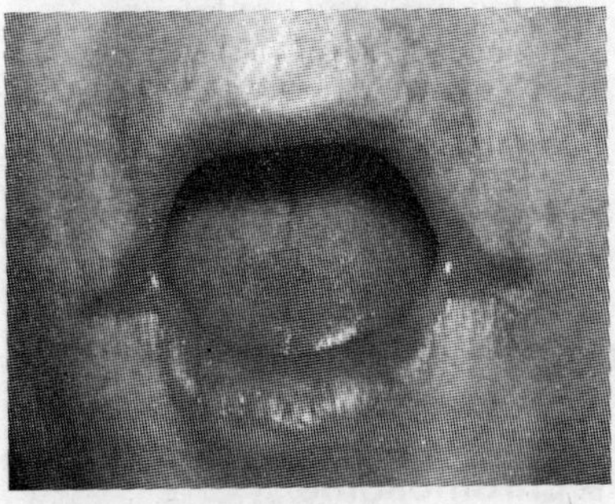

chemokine

a chemical produced by cells that stimulate the activity of other cells. Certain chemokines are associated with autoimmune disorder and some, e.g. MIP-1-alpha, MIP-1-beta, RANTES, have been shown to affect the activity of HIV.

chemoprophylaxis

disease prevention using chemicals.

chemotherapy

the chemical treatment of disease, especially cancer.

chi

see **qi.**

chickenpox

an acute contagious disease caused by the varicella-zoster virus (VZV) and characterised by low-grade fever and a rash of itchy fluid-filled vesicles. Chickenpox typically occurs in children. VZV may reactivate later in life to cause shingles, a painful blistering rash.

Baby with severe chickenpox

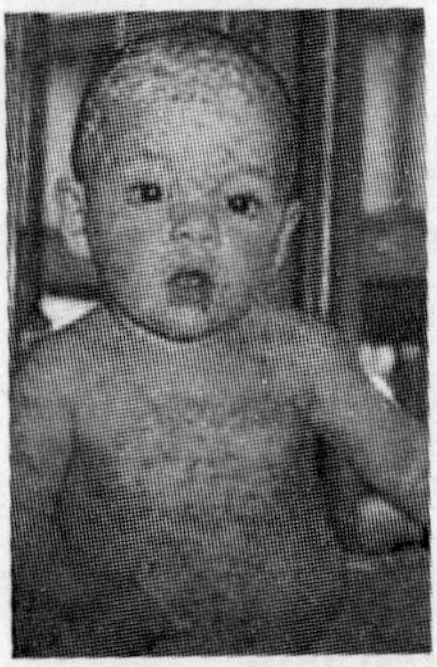

chiropractic

a system of treatment based on the manipulation of the spinal vertebrae, the misalignment of which is believed to be responsible for pain and illness.

chlamydia
a bacterial infection that can cause disease, left untreated it can lead to cancer.

chlamydiasis
an infection, usually sexually transmitted, with the bacteria Chlamydia trachomatis. Chlamydiasis is the most common sexually transmitted disease in the U.S. It may be asymptomatic or include symptoms such as genital inflammation and discharge, pelvic pain and fever. Untreated chlamydiasis may lead to pelvic inflammatory disease (PID) and infertility. Chlamydia may also cause eye disease (trachoma) and pneumonia.

cholangitis
inflammation of the bile ducts, often characterised by jaundice.

cholecystitis
inflammation of the gall bladder, the organ that stores bile.

cholestasis
obstruction of the flow of bile from the gall bladder.

cholesterol
a substance in animal tissue that is an essential component of cell membranes and nerve fibre insulation. Cholesterol is important for the metabolism and transport of fatty acids and in the production of hormones and Vitamin D. Cholesterol is manufactured by the liver and is also present in certain foods (e.g., eggs, shellfish). There are 2 types of cholesterol in the blood, high-density (HDL) and low-density (LDL) lipoproteins. Very low cholesterol levels may indicate malnutrition.

chop
a chemotherapeutic regimen for cancer treatment that combines cyclophosphamide, hydroxyldaunomycin (doxorubicin or Adriamycin), vincristine (Oncovin) and prednisone.

chorion
one of the membranes that encloses the foetus within the uterus.

chorionic gonadotropin
see **human chorionic gonadotropin.**

chromosome
a structure of compact intertwined molecules of DNA found in the nucleus of cells. Chromosome contains the cell's genetic information. Humans normally have 46 chromosomes.

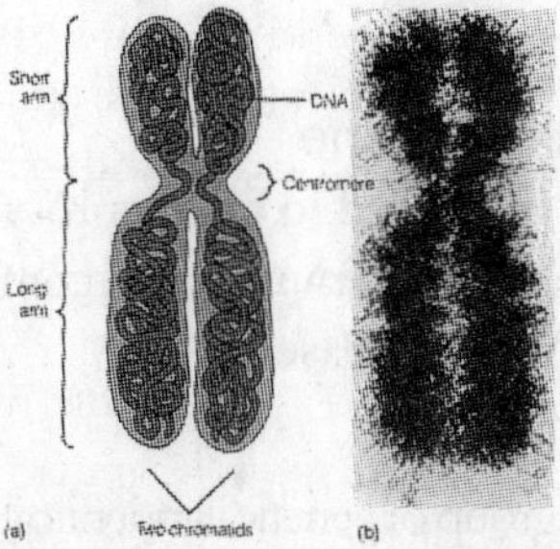

■ **chronic**
continuing, constant, lingering, prolonged.

■ **Chronic Fatigue Syndrome (CFS)**
an illness characterised by fatigue, neurological problems, joint and muscle pain and impairment of the ability to function normally for 6 months or longer. CFS is associated with impaired natural killer cell activity. The cause of CFS is unknown, but the condition may be associated with a virus, e.g. Epstein-Barr virus.

■ **cidofovir**
a nucleoside analog drug used to treat refractory cytomegalovirus (CMV) infection and acyclovir-resistant herpes simplex virus.

■ **cimetidine (tagamet)**
a drug directed against histamine receptors. Cimetidine is used to treat peptic (stomach) ulcers by blocking the secretion of stomach acid and is under study for the treatment of HIV disease.

■ **CIN**
see **cervical intraepithelial neoplasia.**

■ **ciprofloxacin (cipro)**
an oral antibiotic used to treat common bacterial infections and used — in combination with other drugs — to treat Mycobacterium avium complex disease in people with AIDS. Side effects may include gastrointestinal distress, seizures and rash.

■ **cirrhosis**
a condition in which the liver becomes scarred, fibrous and filled with fat, thus reducing its ability to function. Causes include infection, e.g. hepatitis and excessive alcohol consumption.

■ **CKR5 (ccr5, cc-ckr5)**
a protein found on certain blood cells that serves as a receptor site for chemokines. CKR5 acts as a co-receptor, which HIV uses to infect cells. Individuals who lack a functional copy of the gene that makes CKR5 are believed to be non-susceptible to HIV infection.

■ **clade**
see **subtype.**

■ **clarithromycin (biaxin)**
a macrolide antibiotic used to treat

bacterial infections. Clarithromycin is used as treatment and prophylaxis for Mycobacterium avium complex (MAC). Side effects include nausea, taste changes and abdominal pain.

■ **clindamycin (cleocin)**
an antibiotic used as treatment and prophylaxis for toxoplasmosis and treatment of PCP in combination with other drugs.

■ **clinical**
relating to the treatment of patients. A clinical observation is based on the observed condition of patients and their symptoms, as distinguished from blood tests or other laboratory findings.

■ **clinical trial**
a method for testing an experimental drug.

■ **clinical trial (clinical study)**
an organised procedure for determining the effectiveness of a new drug or therapy by administering the agent to participants under strictly controlled conditions. In many clinical trials new agents are tested against older agents or an inactive substance (placebo). The clinical trials process includes Phase I, II and III trials and Phase IV postmarketing evaluation.

■ **clofazimine**
a drug used to treat leprosy and Mycobacterium avium complex (MAC) disease.

■ **clone**
a group of genetically identical cells or organisms derived from a single common ancestor. Also refers to the process of creating identical cells or organisms. Monoclonal refers to the products, e.g. antibodies, of a single clone.

■ **clotrimazole (mycelex)**
an antifungal drug approved as a treatment for candidiasis.

■ **clotting factor**
one of several proteins involved in the normal clotting of blood.

■ **Cluster Differentiation (CD)**
a marker protein embedded in the surface of cell membranes or the interior of cells. CD molecules determine which other molecules can bind to a given cell, e.g. the CD4 marker allows HIV to invade certain types of cells.

■ **CMI**
see **cell-mediated immunity.**

■ **CMV**
abbreviation, cytomegalovirus. One disease caused by this virus

is CMV retinitis, which can cause blindness if left untreated. CMV disease is an AIDS-defining condition.

■ CNS

abbreviation, **Central Nervous System.**

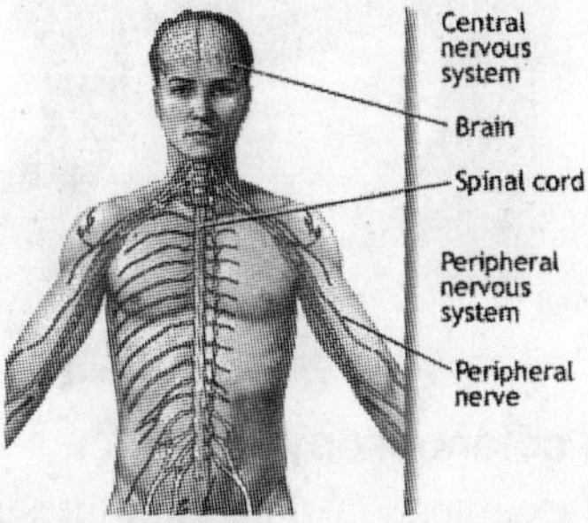

■ co-factor

a factor, e.g. substance, microorganism, environmental condition, that influences the progression of a disease or the action of a disease-causing agent.

■ co-receptor

a second receptor that enables an organism to infect a cell. In addition to the CD4 receptor on cell surfaces, HIV requires the co-receptor fusin to infect T-cells and the co-receptor CKR5 to infect macrophages.

■ coagulation

clotting, the transformation of a liquid (e.g., blood) into a solid mass.

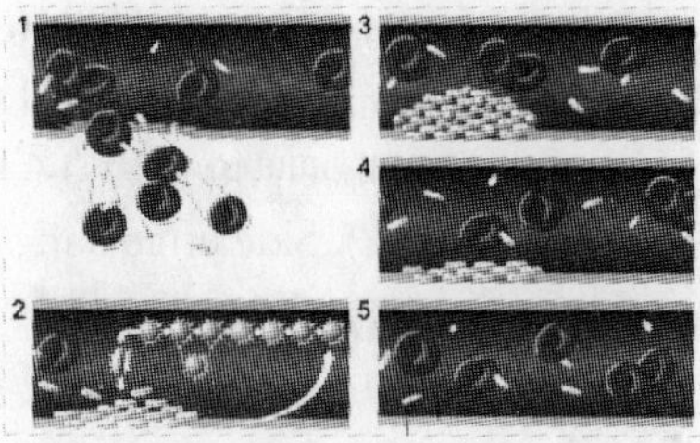

■ cobalamin (vitamin b12)

see **vitamin B**

■ coccidioidomycosis

a fungal disease characterised by fever and localised pulmonary (lung) symptoms. Also called San Joaquin fever. This is considered an AIDS-defining condition.

■ coccidioidomycosis (valley fever)

an uncommon fungal disease acquired by inhaling dust particles containing spores of Coccidioides immitis. The disease is characterised by lesions in the upper respiratory tract and lungs and may sometimes disseminate to visceral organs, bones, skin and other tissues. Symptoms include cough, fatigue, fever and weight loss.

■ codon

a sequence of 3 nucleotides or bases that encodes the information for a particular amino acid (the building blocks that make up proteins). Changes in specific codons can confer resistance to certain drugs (e.g., a codon 215 mutation is associated with AZT resistance).

■ **coenzyme q10 (coq10)**
a quinone substance that facilitates the production of energy from food and acts as an antioxidant.

■ **Cofactor2**
a substance that activates an enzyme, commonly an inorganic ion, coenzyme or vitamin. The virus herpes (HSV) is sometimes called an AIDS cofactor because people infected by both the herpes virus and HIV often progress to AIDS faster than people infected only by HIV.

■ **cognitive impairment**
problems with memory and thinking. Can be caused by HIV. Sometimes used to describe a less severe form of dementia.

■ **cohort**
a group of individuals in a study who share a demographic, clinical or other statistical characteristic, e.g. age, study site.

■ **colitis**
inflammation of the mucous membrane of the colon, which is part of the intestines.

■ **colon**
the large intestine, extending from the cecum, where it meets the small intestine, to the rectum.

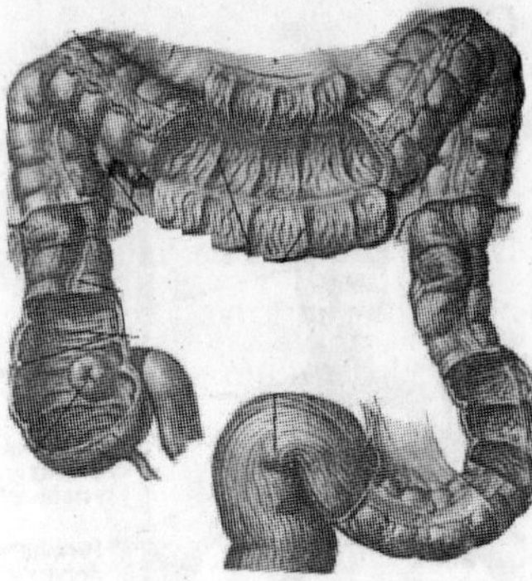

■ **colonoscopy**
examination of the large intestine using a narrow, flexible lighted tube.

■ **Colony-Stimulating Factor (CSF)**
a cytokine responsible for regulating the production of white blood cells. Types include granulocyte colony-stimulating factor (G-CSF) and granulocyte macrophage colony-stimulating factor (GM-CSF), which are used to relieve neutropenia.

■ **colostrum**
breast fluid (produced prior to milk production) that contains large amounts of proteins, calories, immunoglobulins and lymphocytes.

■ colposcopy (biomicroscopy)
examination of a tissue surface (particularly the uterine cervix) with a low-powered, lighted microscope (colposcope) to identify abnormal cell growth and, if necessary, remove a tissue sample for biopsy.

■ combination therapy
using 2, 3 or more drugs at the same time. Studies have shown that taking multiple anti-HIV drugs is more potent than taking a single drug.

■ commensal organism
an organism that normally lives within the body, usually without causing illness.

■ Community Advisory Board (CAB)
a group of community members, e.g., people with HIV/AIDS, care providers, advocates who provide recommendations regarding clinical research.

■ Community Constituency Group (CCG)
a group of individuals representing diverse communities affected by HIV/AIDS that advises the ACTG on issues related to clinical research.

■ Community Programs For Clinical Research On Aids (CPCRA)
a community-based clinical trials network sponsored by NIAID. CPCRA conducts Phase II and III studies in community settings with a focus on new treatments for opportunistic infections, particularly in underserved populations.

■ Community-Based Organisation (CBO)
a local organisation within a community that provides various services to people with HIV/AIDS.

■ compartment
a separate structural portion, e.g. of the body or of a cell. The term is also used in pharmacology to denote an area of the body where a drug is metabolised, but which may not have a discrete physical boundary.

■ compassionate use
a classification of an experimental drug (IND) that is made available to seriously ill patients before the drug is approved for general use. Few drugs get this classification. Compassionate use drugs are usually free to the patient.

■ complement
proteins in the blood that play a part in immune defence against

invading organisms. Complement proteins, in conjunction with an antibody-antigen complex, initiate a sequence of events — the complement cascade — that results in the destruction of the membrane of the organism or cell under attack.

■ complementary therapy

an additional treatment or therapy that adds benefit to an existing treatment regimen.

■ Complete Blood Count (CBC)

a screening of the cellular components of the blood, including red blood cell count including hematocrit and haemoglobin, counts of various types of white blood cells such as granulocytes and T-cells and platelet count.

■ compliance

adherence by a patient to a prescribed medical regimen.

■ compound q

see **trichosanthin.**

■ Computed Tomography Scan (CT scan)

a method of visualising soft tissues of the body using X-rays. Also known as computed axial tomography or CAT scan.

■ concomitant

accompanied by or occurring at the same time. Concomitant therapies are those that are used together.

■ concurrent

occurring at (or, for drugs, taken at) the same time.

■ condom

a sheath made of latex, polyurethane or animal membrane that is worn over the penis to prevent transmission of semen. Condoms are used to prevent pregnancy. Latex and polyurethane condoms protect against the spread of HIV and other sexually transmitted diseases.

■ condylomata acuminata

genital and/or anal warts caused by infection with a strain of the human papillomavirus (HPV). Warts may appear as tiny white spots or as larger tumours or masses. Condylomata acuminata is typically sexually transmitted and may be particularly aggressive in people with HIV disease (e.g., increased number and size of warts, more frequent recurrence). Warts may be treated with chemicals, surgery or cryotherapy (freezing).

■ **cone biopsy (conization)**
removal of a cone-shaped wedge from the bottom of the uterine cervix to remove lesions and to provide a tissue sample for biopsy.

■ **confidence level (confidence interval)**
a statistical measure of the likelihood that an experimental result is 'real' and not the result of chance alone. Confidence improves as larger numbers of participants are included in a trial.

■ **confounder**
a factor that can influence a trial or experiment, leading to unexpected outcomes that improperly skew the results.

■ **congenital**
refers to a disease or condition that is present from the time of birth.

■ **conjunctivitis (pink eye)**
inflammation of the conjunctiva, the membrane that covers the eyeball, characterised by redness, watering and itching.

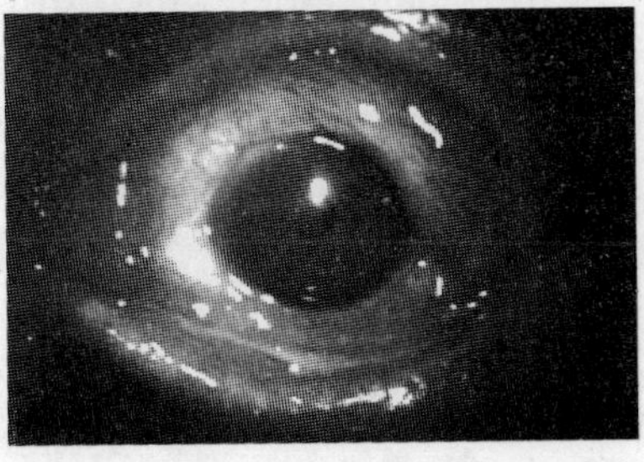

■ **constitutional**
not local, affecting the whole body. Constitutional symptoms of HIV disease include fever and night sweats.

■ **contact tracing**
a method of finding and informing persons who may have contracted an infectious disease, e.g., through sexual or needle-sharing contact with a person known to be HIV positive.

■ **contagious**
a disease that may be transmitted by casual contact from one person to another, e.g. through droplets in the air, on the hands.

■ **contraception**
birth control. A contraceptive is an agent or method that prevents conception or successful gestation.

■ **contraindication**
any circumstance or condition that makes a method of treatment inadvisable in a particular case.

■ **control arm**
a comparison group in a scientific experiment, e.g. a clinical drug trial that is used to verify experimental results. A control group is not subject to the intervention under, e.g. not given a

drug so that those receiving the intervention and those not receiving it may be compared. Contrast with treatment arm.

■ controlled trial
a clinical trial in which the group receiving an experimental therapy is compared to a control group that is not given the intervention being studied. In a placebo-controlled trial, the control group is given an inactive substance i.e. placebo. In an active control trial the control group is given the best existing proven therapy. Contrast with uncontrolled trial.

■ convergent therapy
a regimen consisting of several drugs aimed at the same structural or functional target (e.g. a combination of 3 reverse transcriptase inhibitors).

■ cord blood
blood taken from the remains of the umbilical cord after birth. Cord blood is rich in stem cells.

■ core
the internal portion of the HIV viral particle. The core proteins, encoded by the gag gene, include the glycoproteins p24 and p17.

■ corroborate
to confirm.

■ cortex (adjective cortical)
the outer part of an organ, e.g. cerebral cortex, adrenal cortex.

■ corticosteroid
one of a group of steroid hormones, e.g., prednisone, corticosterone, cortisone, aldosterone) produced by the cortex of the adrenal gland or manufactured synthetically. Corticosteroids are used in the treatment of a variety of conditions. They have anti-inflammatory and immunosuppressive properties.

■ cortisol
a steroid hormone secreted by the adrenal cortex as part of the body's response to stress. Cortisol promotes the breakdown of body tissues to provide energy and raw materials, high cortisol levels are associated with reduced immune function. Synthetic cortisol (hydrocortisone) is used to reduce inflammation and lessen allergic reactions.

■ cost recovery
a program under which drug companies are paid to provide a new drug at the expanded access stage, before marketing approval has been granted.

Community Programs For Clinical Research On Aids (CPCRA)

a network of primary care physicians and nurses who work with NIAID staff to design and conduct community-based clinical trials in patients with HIV disease and AIDS.

creatinine

a protein, a normal metabolic waste product found in muscles and blood. The amount of creatinine in the blood or urine tells doctors how well your kidneys are working.

Creatinine Phosphokinase (CPK)

an enzyme essential for muscle contraction. Blood levels of CPK are typically elevated in muscle diseases (myopathies) and CPK levels can be used to monitor toxicity to the muscles.

crixivan

brand name of indinavir.

crohn's disease

a type of enteritis or inflammation of the intestines.

cross-immunity

a state in which immunity to one organism serves to protect an individual against a different but related organism, e.g., immunity against cowpox provides immunity against smallpox.

cross-reactivity

a process by which an antibody responds to an antigen other than that which originally stimulated its production.

cross-resistance

the development of resistance to one agent, e.g. a drug, which also confers resistance to another agent, e.g. a similar drug of the same class.

cross-tolerance

a situation in which tolerance to one drug carries over to another related drug, so that the similar drug has reduced effects.

crossover

a trial design in which the therapy given to different arms is switched during the course of the trial, e.g. the arm receiving drug is switched to placebo and vice-versa.

cryotherapy

1. treatment procedure involving intense cold, e.g. freezing genital warts.

2. the use of liquid nitrogen to freeze an abnormal lesion; the lesion typically forms a blister and then heals. Cryotherapy is sometimes used to induce scar

formation in order to prevent further spread of abnormal cells, e.g. in cases of cervical dysplasia or retinitis.

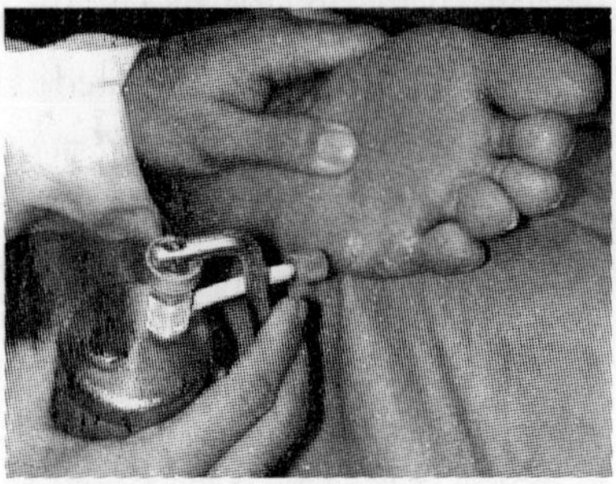

■ cryptococcal meningitis

a fungal infection of the brain and spinal cord. Symptoms include severe headache, dizziness, nausea, weight loss, vision disorders and mental deterioration. Meningitis with headache, blurred vision, confusion, dizziness, nausea, anorexia, depression, agitation or slurred speech are other common symptoms.

■ cryptococcosis

an infection caused by a yeast-like fungus, typically Cryptococcus neoformans, found in soil and bird faeces. A common manifestation is cryptococcal meningitis (CM), an inflammation of the membranes surrounding the brain and spinal cord. Cryptococcosis may also become disseminated. Symptoms may include nausea, fever, headache, dizziness, stiff neck, vision and speech difficulties, changes in mental status, increased intracranial pressure and seizures. Untreated CM can lead to coma and death. Cryptococcosis may also affect the lungs and may become disseminated, resulting in a red skin rash. Treatments include oral fluconazole and amphotericin B.

■ cryptosporidiosis

an infection whose main symptom is prolonged diarrhoea which leads to weight loss. All treatments for this illness are still experimental.

■ CTL

Cytotoxic T Lymphocyte. A cell that kills foreign cells that were marked for destruction by other immune system cells. The immune systems' hit squad.

■ culture

a method of growing a microorganism or living tissue in vitro in a medium that promotes its growth.

■ cunnilingus

oral sex on a woman. Sexual contact between one person's tongue and/or mouth and a woman's vulva, clitoris and/or vagina.

■ **curcumin**
an compound present in the spice turmeric. Curcumin has anti-inflammatory and antioxidant properties and is under study as an anti-HIV therapy.

■ **custodial care**
care that provides for daily needs and bodily maintenance, e.g. feeding, hygiene rather than attempting to provide a cure.

■ **cutaneous**
pertaining to the skin.

■ **cyanosis**
a dark purplish coloration of the skin and mucous membranes due to deficient oxygen in the blood.

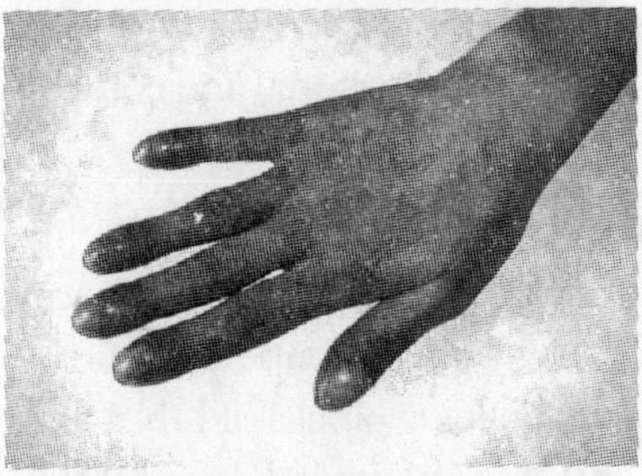

■ **cyclooxygenase**
an enzyme involved in oxygen metabolism. Cyclooxygenase is part of the pathway that mediates bodily response to infection and injury, e.g. inflammation and pain via substances such as histamine and prostaglandins.

■ **cyclospora**
an intestinal parasite that can cause severe diarrhoea in people with AIDS. A recent outbreak was associated with contaminated North American strawberries.

■ **Cyclosporin A**
a drug that suppresses the immune system. The drug is commonly used in organ transplant recipients to prevent tissue or organ rejection.

■ **cyst**
a stage in the life cycle of certain parasites, during which they are enclosed within a protective wall. Anti-parasitic drugs often have no effect against cysts.

■ **cysteine**
a sulphur-bearing amino acid that makes up part of the compound glutathione.

■ **cystitis**
an inflammation of the urinary bladder.

■ **cyto-**
prefix, cell.

■ **Cytochrome P450 System**
a process that metabolises drugs and other foreign substances in the liver, by means of the CP450 enzymes.

■ cytokine
protein produced by some white blood cells (macrophages, monocytes, lymphocytes) used as messengers. Cytokinds produced in the lymph system are also called lymphokinds.

■ cytology
the study of the structure, function and pathology of cells.

■ cytolytic
having a destructive effect on cells, causing them to erupt or burst.

■ cytomegalovirus
abbreviation, cytomegalovirus. One disease caused by this virus is CMV retinitis, which can cause blindness if left untreated. CMV disease is an AIDS-defining condition, commonly abbreviated CMV.

■ cytomegalovirus (CMV, human herpesvirus 5)
a herpes virus. CMV infection often occurs in healthy individuals without causing symptoms. In immuno-compromised individuals (usually at CD4 counts below 50 cells/mm3), CMV may cause serious illness including retinitis (inflammation of the retina), pneumonia, colitis (inflammation of the large bowel) and encephalitis. CMV infection of a pregnant woman may lead to congenital abnormalities in the newborn. CMV may be treated with ganciclovir, foscarnet or cidofovir.

■ cytopathogenicity
ability to cause disease in cells.

■ cytopathology
disease, disorders or destruction of cells.

■ cytopenia
reduced levels of the cellular elements in the blood.

■ cytoplasm
the gel-like substance that composes cells and lies outside the cell nucleus. The cytoplasm contains numerous structures or organelles (e.g., mitochondria) and component substances.

■ cytosine (c)
one of the pyrimidine nucleic acid bases that make up nucleotides, the building blocks of DNA and RNA. The antiviral drug, DDI is a nucleoside analog associated with cytosine.

■ Cytotoxic T-Lymphocyte (CTL, T-Killer Cell)
a type of white blood cell that bears the CD8 surface marker and targets and kills cells infected with viruses, bacteria, parasites and other

micro-organisms. The action of CTL is coordinated by CD4 cells via the production of cytokines. The immune system's hit squad.

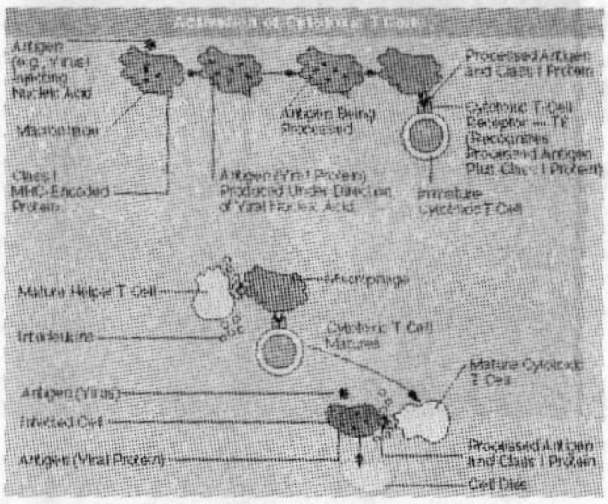

■ cytotoxicity (adjective cytotoxic)

the quality of being toxic to or killing cells.

■ cytotoxin

a protein poisonous to certain cells.

■ cytovene

brand name of ganciclovir. D D4T (STAVUDINE, ZERIT): an antiviral nucleoside analog drug approved for the treatment of HIV disease. D4T inhibits the activity of the reverse transcriptase enzyme needed for HIV replication. Side effects include nausea, peripheral neuropathy and liver toxicity.

■ d.t.d.no.

pharmaceutical abbreviation, give doses (dentur talis doses numus).

■ dapsone

an antibiotic drug used in the treatment and prophylaxis of PCP. Side effects may include nausea, dizziness, skin rash, photosensitivity and anaemia.

■ Data Safety And Monitoring Board (DSMB)

a group of experts that evaluates clinical trials for safety and ethics. DSMB typically examines interim data as a trial progresses and determines whether it should be stopped or allowed to continue.

■ daunorubicin

a chemotherapeutic drug used to treat Kaposi's sarcoma and other cancers.

■ daunoxome

a liposomal (fat bubble) formulation of daunorubicin that allows more precise targeting of the drug with fewer side effects.

■ DDC (zalcitabine, dideoxycytidine, hivid)

a nucleoside analog drug that inhibits HIV replication by interfering with the reverse transcriptase enzyme. The drug is approved for the treatment of HIV disease; current practice favours use in combinations. Adverse side effects may include nausea, peripheral neuropathy oral ulcers and pancreatitis.

DDI (didanosine, dideoxyinosine, videx)
a nucleoside analog drug that inhibits HIV replication. The drug is approved for the treatment of HIV disease; current practice favours use in combinations. Side effects may include diarrhoea, pancreatitis and peripheral neuropathy.

deferred therapy
therapy given later in the course of disease, often after symptoms have appeared. In a clinical trial, one arm may be given deferred treatment and compared to an arm that received treatment from the outset.

definitive
conclusive, unquestionable. A definitive diagnosis is made by detection of an organism (e.g., virus, bacteria) via culture, biopsy or other procedure.

degenerative
relating to a progressive deterioration of a tissue or organ leading to structural or functional impairment.

dehydration
loss or lack of water in the body. Dehydration may result from prolonged vomitting or diarrhoea and may interfere with or disrupt many bodily processes.

Dehydroepiandrosterone (DHEA)
a weak androgenic steroid produced by the adrenal cortex. DHEA levels are often decreased in people with HIV disease.

delavirdine (rescriptor)
a non-nucleoside reverse transcriptase inhibitor drug.

Delayed-Type Hypersensitivity (DTH)
a cell-mediated immune response that peaks 24-72 hours after restimulation with an antigen to which the body has previously been exposed. In an antigen skin test, a local DTH reaction characterised by redness and induration (hardness and swelling) may be seen.

delirium
a state of mental confusion, typically acute and rapid in onset, It may be caused by factors including disease, drug use and high fever.

delta study
a large European clinical trial, with sites in the UK, Germany, France, Italy, the Netherlands, Switzerland and Australia, that compared anti-HIV regimens and determined that combination therapy produced the best results.

■ **Delta-9 Tetrahydrocannabinol**

the active ingredient in marijuana. THC has psychoactive properties, may induce euphoria and drowsiness and may improve appetite and reduce nausea due to chemotherapy.

■ **dementia**

deterioration of intellectual faculties, often accompanied by emotional disturbance. HIV is active in the brain (central nervous system) and can cause dementia, even in those with high CD4 counts and low viral loads. Treatment usually involves an anti-HIV drug — such as AZT — that is able to cross the blood-brain barrier, also called ADC.

■ **demodex folliculorum**

mites that inhabit the skin and are usually found in the sebaceous glands and hair follicles. Although the mites are present and do not cause symptoms in most people, they may cause clusters of tiny bumps in immuno-suppressed people.

■ **demographics**

the characteristics of a population, e.g., sex, race, age, geographic location.

■ **demyelinating neuropathy**

a type of nerve damage that involves demyelination, the loss of the lipid myelin sheath that surrounds nerve cells.

■ **demyelination**

destruction or loss of the myelin (a fatty substance) sheath that surrounds and insulates the axons of nerve cells and is necessary for the proper conduction of neural impulses.

■ **dendritic cell**

a type of immune system cell with many branches. Dendritic cells are found in the skin and mucosal membranes. They are typically the first to arrive at sites of injury or infection, where they bind to invaders and transport them to the lymph nodes where the cell-mediated immune response is initiated. Dendritic cells carry the CD4 surface marker and may be among the first cells to be infected by HIV.

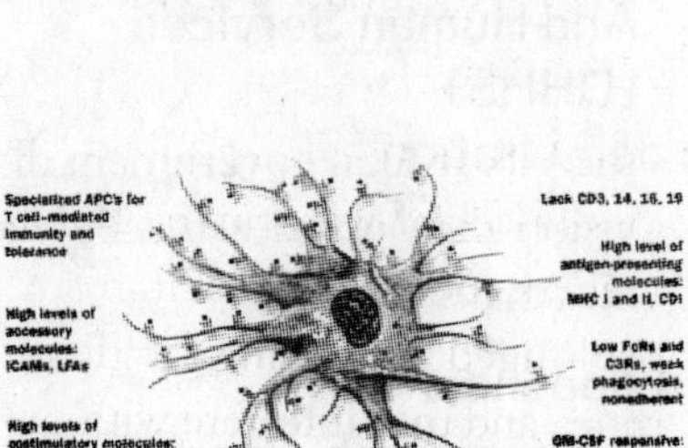

dental dam (latex dam)
a flat latex square, traditionally used for dental surgery, that can be used to protect against the transmission of HIV and other sexually-transmitted diseases. A dental dam (or a substitute such as plastic wrap) is placed between the mouth of one partner and the genitals or anus of another, thus preventing the exchange of fluids during oral sexual contact.

Deoxyribonucleic Acid (DNA)
a molecule found in the nucleus of cells as a twisted double-stranded chain that encodes genetic information. The particular sequence of 4 chemical building blocks (nucleotides) — adenine, cytosine, guanine and thymine — that make up a DNA chain determines the unique genetic code of an individual. See also ribonucleic acid.

Department Of Health And Human Services (DHHS)
the U.S. federal government division that includes the Public Health Service.

dependence
a state in which a person is reliant on a drug. Physical dependence is characterised by the onset of physical symptoms of withdrawal (e.g., sweating, tremors) if a drug is abruptly stopped. Psychological dependence (addiction) is a psychological syndrome characterised by drug craving, compulsive use and relapse after abstinence.

depo-provera
a form of progesterone injected intramuscularly for contraception.

depot form
a method of drug administration in which a drug is injected into a muscle or beneath the skin and slowly absorbed over a period of time, resulting in sustained action.

dermal
relating to the skin.

dermatitis
inflammation of the skin.

dermatology
the medical specialty concerned with diseases and disorders of the skin.

dermatophytosis
an infection caused by dermatophytes, a type of fungal organism. Tinea pedis (athlete's foot)

and tinea cruris (jock itch) are forms of dermatophytosis.

- **desensitisation**
  the reduction of sensitivity or allergic reaction to an antigen or a drug, typically achieved by administering a small amount and gradually increasing the dose.

- **dexamethasone**
  a steroid with anti-inflammatory properties.

- **DHEA**
  see **dehydroepiandrosterone.**

- **diabetes**
  a disease characterised by excessive urination. Diabetes mellitus is caused by insufficient insulin production or lack of responsiveness to insulin, resulting in hyperglycaemia (high blood glucose levels). There are 2 primary types of diabetes mellitus, type I (insulin-dependent or juvenile-onset), which may be caused by an autoimmune response and type II (non-insulin-dependent or adult-onset). Diabetes insipidus is typically due to hormonal dysregulation.

- **diagnosis**
  the determination of the existence of a disease or condition. Diagnosis generally involves the evaluation of a patient's medical history, clinical symptoms and laboratory test results.

- **dialysis**
  a procedure for cleansing the blood using membranes to filter out waste elements. Kidney dialysis is used to substitute for the function of damaged or absent kidneys.

- **diaphragm**
  a flexible sheet. The diaphragm in the chest is a sheet of muscle that controls breathing. Also refers to a flexible latex disk placed over the uterine cervix, as a contraceptive device to form a barrier to sperm.

- **diarrhoea**
  frequent, loose bowel movements. Diarrhoea may be caused by a variety of factors including bacteria (e.g., Mycobacterium avium, Salmonella), viruses (e.g., CMV), parasites (e.g., Cryptosporidium parvum, Giardia) and drug use. Persistent diarrhoea is common in persons with HIV disease and may lead to wasting due to inadequate nutrient absorption.

- **Diethylhomospermine (DEHSPM)**
  an experimental, non-opiate, anti-diarrhoea drug, that delays intes-

tinal transit and enhances fluid absorption.

■ **dietician**
a person specialising in dietetics, the study of nutrition and the use of special diets for prophylaxis and treatment of disease.

■ **differential diagnosis**
a method of diagnosis that involves determining from a list of possible diseases which is the probable cause of a patient's symptoms, often by a process of elimination.

■ **diffuse**
spread out; not concentrated.

■ **Directly Observed Therapy (Dot)**
a method of medication administration in which a health care provider or other observer watches the patient take each drug dose. DOT is most commonly used for tuberculosis treatment.

■ **discordant**
not having the same serostatus, for example a couple in which one partner is HIV positive and the other is HIV negative.

■ **disseminate**
to spread. A disseminated infection is one that is distributed throughout the body, possibly causing symptoms at multiple sites.

■ **distal**
farthest from the centre or from a central point of reference.

■ **Distal Symmetrical Polyneuropathy (DSPN)**
a common type of peripheral neuropathy in people with HIV disease characterised by pain, burning or tingling sensations, weakness and/or numbness, especially in the hands and feet.

■ **disulfiram (antabuse)**
a drug used in the treatment of alcoholism. Alcohol consumption causes nausea in people taking disulfiram. The drug is similar to DTC (Imuthiol), an experimental AIDS treatment.

■ **diuretic**
an agent that increases the amount of urine excreted.

■ **diurnal**
twice a day.

■ **DNCB**
dinitrochlorobenzene, a solvent chemical. Some believe that the use of DNCB on the skin provokes a generalised immune system response.

■ **dosage (dose)**
the amount of a substance, e.g. a drug that is given at one time.

■ **dosage regimen**
a formalised schedule by which drugs are administered, including the amount of drug, the number of doses per time period and the time between doses.

■ **dose**
a specified quantity of a drug, prescribed to be taken at a specified interval.

■ **dose escalation**
the gradual increase of drug dosages to determine the amount that delivers the best balance of high efficacy and few side effects. Dose-escalation trials are clinical studies that monitor the effects of increasing dosages of a drug.

■ **dose escalation trial**
a clinical trial involving volunteers who take escalating amounts of a drug. Researchers are looking for the largest quantity of the substance that can be tolerated without an adverse reaction.

■ **dose ranging trial**
a clinical trial involving groups of volunteers given different quantities of a substance (or the same quantity but at different intervals). Results of the groups are compared to find which quantities and intervals give the best results and produce the fewest adverse reactions.

■ **dose-ranging**
a clinical trial in which different doses of a drug are compared to determine which dosage has the best balance of high efficacy and low toxicity.

■ **dose-response relationship**
a phenomenon by which increased doses of a drug lead to increased effects, such that the response to a drug is directly related to the dose administered.

■ **dot**
pharmaceutical abbreviation, direct observational therapy.

■ **double-blind**
a type of clinical trial in which neither the subject nor the investigator knows what treatment, if any, the subject is receiving. At the end of the trial the 'code' is broken and data are analysed. Double-blinding is done to minimize bias due to the expectations of the subject, investigator(s) and/or healthcare provider(s).

■ **double-blind trial**
a clinical trial involving volunteers who take an experimental drug

or a control substance. The control substance is usually a drug already approved for use in the disease, but sometimes it's a placebo. In a double-blind trial, a lab prepares the experimental and control substances and labels them so that neither the researchers nor patients know which individuals are getting the experimental drug. Only after the trial is finished do the researchers and patients learn which patients were taking the experimental drug. In HIV-related trials, the placebo is commonly replaced with some approved anti-HIV treatment. (also see clinical trial and open label trial.).

■ **downregulation**
reduction of the rate at which a process occurs, a substance is released, etc.

■ **doxorubicin (adriamycin)**
an anti-cancer drug used to treat leukaemia, lymphoma, Kaposi's sarcoma and other malignancies. Side effects include mouth sores and bone marrow suppression.

■ **dox-sl (doxil)**
a formulation of doxorubicin encapsulated in liposomes (fat bubbles).

■ **dronabinol**
a synthetic version of THC, the active agent in marijuana. Dronabinol is used to reduce nausea and vomitting caused by chemotherapy and as an appetite stimulant in people with wasting syndrome. Side effects may include drowsiness, confusion and coordination difficulties.

■ **droplet nuclei**
airborne particles that transmit infection (e.g. tuberculosis).

■ **drug interaction**
a change in the way one drug acts when it is taken with some other drug or substance. Also called drug interaction.

■ **DSMB**
see **Data and Safety Monitoring Board.**

■ **duodenum (adjective duodenal)**
the first part of the small intestine where it meets the stomach.

■ **dys-**
prefix, abnormal, often used to mean difficult or painful.

■ **dysmenorrhea**
difficult or painful menstruation (e.g. cramps).

■ **dyspareunia**
painful sexual intercourse.

■ **dysphagia**
difficult or painful swallowing.

■ **dysplasia**
abnormal tissue or cell growth.

■ **dyspnoea**
difficult, laboured breathing; shortness of breath.

■ **dysregulation**
interruption of or interference with the normal processes.

■ **dysthymia**
a chronic mood disorder, characterised by depression.

■ **dystrophy**
progressive tissue changes. Several dystrophic diseases (e.g., muscular dystrophy) are characterised by muscle wasting and dysfunction.

■ **e.m.p.**
pharmaceutical abbreviation, in the manner prescribed (*ex modo praescripto*).

■ **ebv**
abbreviation, Epstein-Barr virus.

■ **ectopic pregnancy**
a pregnancy in which a fertilised egg begins to develop outside the uterus (e.g., in a fallopian tube). Ectopic pregnancy can lead to tubal rupture, haemorrhage and death.

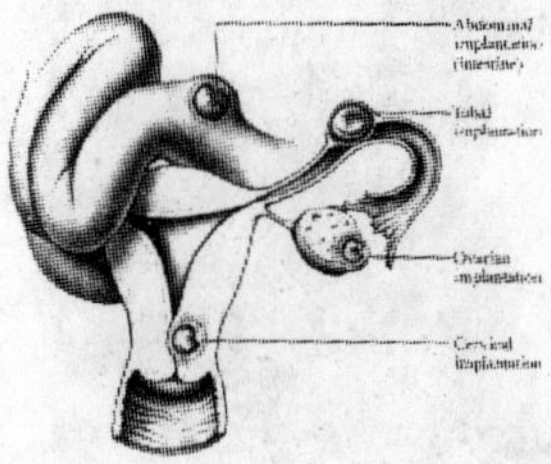

Ectopic Pregnancy

■ **eczema**
an acute or chronic inflammatory condition of the skin.

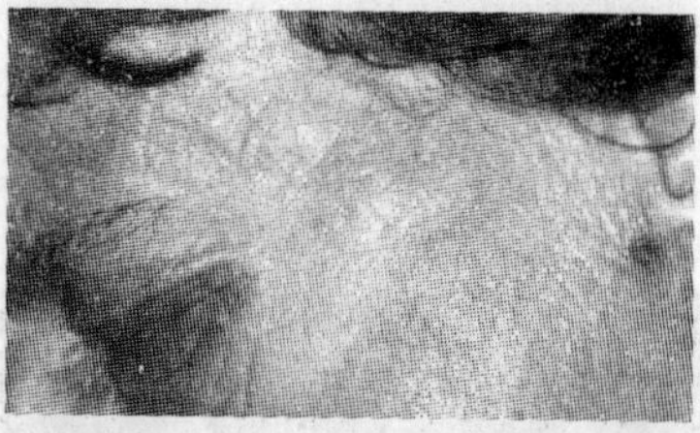

■ **EEG**
see **Electroencephalography.**

■ **Effective Concentration (EC)**
see **inhibitory concentration.**

■ **efferent**
refers to nerves that travel from the brain and spinal cord to the rest of the body. Contrast with afferent.

■ **efficacy**
effectiveness, the ability to achieve a desired effect.

■ **Electrocardiography (EKG)**
a method of recording the electrical activity of the heart.

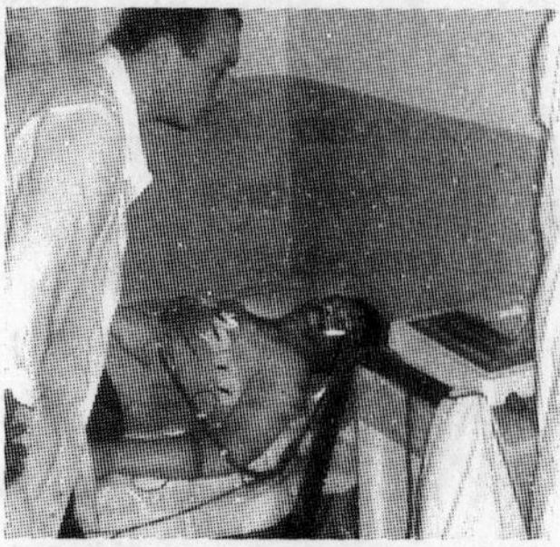

■ **electrocautery (electrodessication)**
a method of destroying lesions or tissue and sealing off blood vessels using a high frequency electric current.

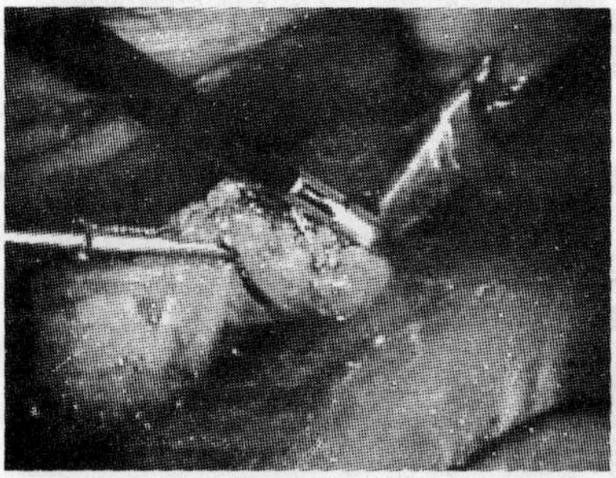

■ **Electroencephalography (EEG)**
a method of recording brain activity using an electroencephalograph, a device which records electrical current.

■ **electrolyte**
an electrically charged element or compound (e.g., sodium, potassium) found in body fluids, tissues and cells. An imbalance of electrolytes can result from prolonged vomitting or diarrhoea and may lead to the disruption of many bodily processes, possibly resulting in muscle weakness, cramps or seizures.

■ **elisa**
a test to see if the patient is HIV positive. The term stands for Enzyme-Linked Immunosorbent Assay.

■ **empiric diagnosis/treatment (presumptive diagnosis)**
evaluation and/or treatment based on observation and experience alone, without relying on laboratory test results or while awaiting laboratory results.

■ **encephalitis**
inflammation of the brain.

■ **encephalopathy**
a disease of the brain. This infection is considered as an AIDS-defining condition.

■ **endemic**
the continuous presence of a disease in a geographic location, community or population.

■ **endo-**
Prefix, internal, inside or originating from within the body or an organ.

■ **endocarditis**
inflammation of the inner membranes of the heart.

■ **endocrine gland**
a ductless gland that regulates body functions via hormones secreted into the bloodstream. The endocrine system includes the hypothalamus, pituitary gland, thyroid, adrenal glands and gonads (ovaries and testes). Contrast with exocrine gland.

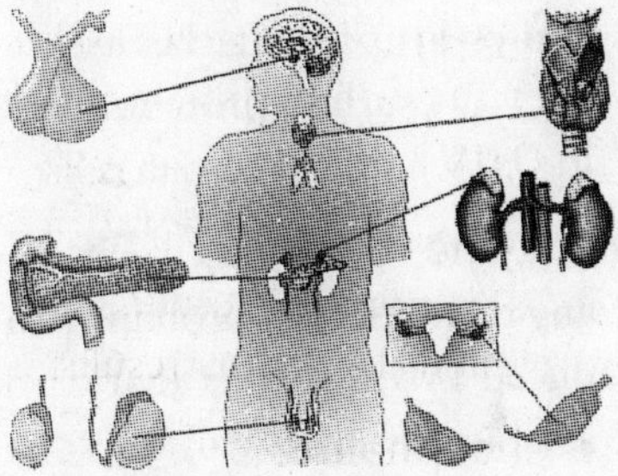

■ **endogenous**
originating within or produced by the body.

■ **endometriosis**
the presence of endometrial tissue outside the uterus, often in the form of cysts. The tissue reacts to hormones and symptoms (primarily pain) typically occur in monthly cycles.

■ **endometrium**
the mucous membrane that lines the uterus.

■ **endorphin**
a group of endogenous (produced by the body) hormones (e.g., beta endorphin, metenkephalin) that are chemically similar to opiate drugs. Endorphins are involved in coping with acute stress and modulating the perception of pain. They may also have a role in mobilising the immune system.

■ **endorphinergic**
inducing or enhancing endorphin production and/or activity.

■ **endoscopy (*adjective* endoscopic)**
a method of examining the interior of a body cavity or hollow organ (e.g. oesophagus, stomach) using an endoscope, a narrow, flexible fibre optic instrument that conducts light.

■ **endothelium (*adjective* endothelial)**
a layer of cells that lines blood and lymph vessels, the heart and various body cavities.

■ **endotoxin**
see **lipopolysaccharide.**

■ **endpoint**
a direct marker of disease progression, e.g., disease symptoms or death. The effectiveness of drug therapies is often deter-

mined by observing the clinical endpoints that develop over time in patients undergoing experimental treatment. Contrast with surrogate marker.

■ **engraftment**
transplantation, the transfer of tissue or an organ from one individual to another.

■ **enhancing antibody**
an antibody that enhances or promotes, rather than inhibits, disease progression. Contrast with neutralising antibody.

■ **entamoeba histolytica**
a parasitic species of amoeba that causes disease in humans. The amoeba invades the bowel mucosa, causing bloody diarrhoea and ulceration, it may also be carried to other organs via the bloodstream. Transmission is by contaminated water oral-anal contact or hand-to-mouth transfer of faecal material.

■ **enteral**
within or by way of the intestines or the gastrointestinal tract.

■ **enteric**
relating to the intestines (e.g., an enteric parasite).

■ **enteritis**
inflammation of the intestines, especially the small intestine.

■ **env**
the gene of HIV that encodes the proteins of the viral envelope, also refers to the proteins produced by the gene.

■ **envelope**
the outer covering of a virus. The HIV envelope contains spikes and is composed of 2 protein subunits, gp120 and gp41, encoded by the env gene. The glycoprotein gp120 attaches itself to the CD4 surface protein, allowing HIV to infect certain cells.

■ **enzyme**
any of numerous proteins produced by organisms that work as a biochemical catalyst.

■ **Enzyme-Linked Immunosorbent Assay (ELISA)**
a laboratory test used to detect the presence of antibodies in the serum. ELISA is used for first-line screening for HIV antibodies. A positive result indicates that antibodies have been detected. The test is sensitive but not specific and a positive ELISA is typically confirmed using a Western Blot assay.

■ **eosinophil**
a leukocyte (blood cell) that can accept eosin stain.

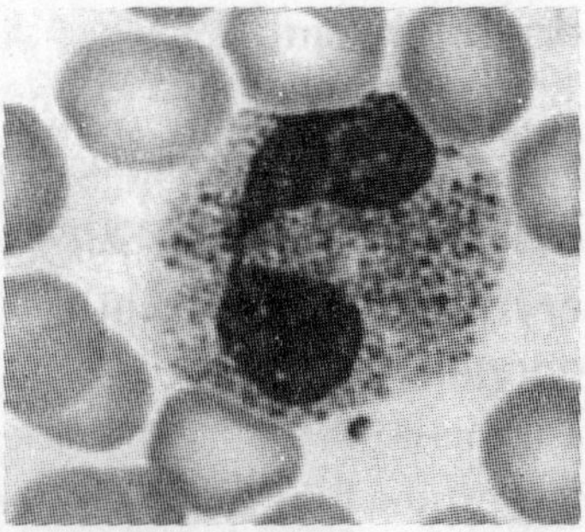

■ **eosinophilia**
increased numbers of eosinophils in the blood characteristic of allergic reactions.

■ **eosinophilic folliculitis**
a rash of itchy, red, pus-filled bumps on the face, arms, chest and back. The cause is unknown, but has been associated with Demodex mites and Pityrosporum yeast. The presence of eosinophils in the hair follicles indicates that the condition may involve an allergic reaction.

■ **epidemic**
an outbreak of a disease within a population.

■ **epidemiology**
the study of the frequency, distribution and behaviour of a disease within a population.

■ **epidermis**
the outer layers of the skin.

■ **epidural**
relating to or administered via the dura mater, the outer membrane of the brain and spinal cord.

■ **epinephrine**
see **adrenaline.**

■ **epithelium**
a thin layer of cells that covers the internal and external surfaces of the body, including body cavities, ducts and vessels.

■ **epitope**
a unique shape or a marker on the surface of an antigen that triggers an antibody response.

■ **Epstein-Barr Virus**
a virus that causes mononucleosis.

■ **Epstein-Barr Virus (EBV, human herpes virus 4)**
a herpesvirus. EBV infection is common and usually asymptomatic in children and may cause infectious mononucleosis ('kissing disease') in young adults. EBV lies dormant in the lymph nodes. It is associated with oral hairy leukoplakia, lymphoid interstitial pneumonitis and some types of cancer in people with suppressed immune systems.

■ **eradication**
the complete elimination of an organism (e.g., HIV) from the

body, including the blood and reservoir tissue sites.

■ erythema (erythematous)
red, especially an inflammatory redness of the skin.

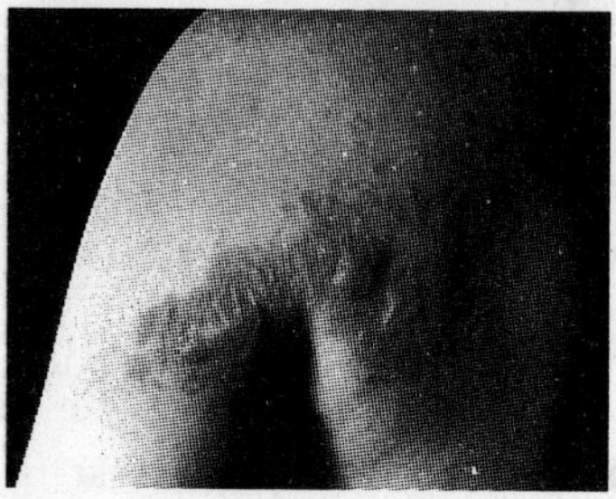

■ erythrocyte
the yellowish disk-shaped blood cell containing haemoglobin. Erythrocytes transport oxygen and carbon dioxide between the lungs and the tissues of the body and are responsible for the colour of blood.

■ erythrocyte sedimentation rate (esr, sed rate)
a blood test that measures the speed at which red blood cells settle in a test tube. The test is used to detect inflammation.

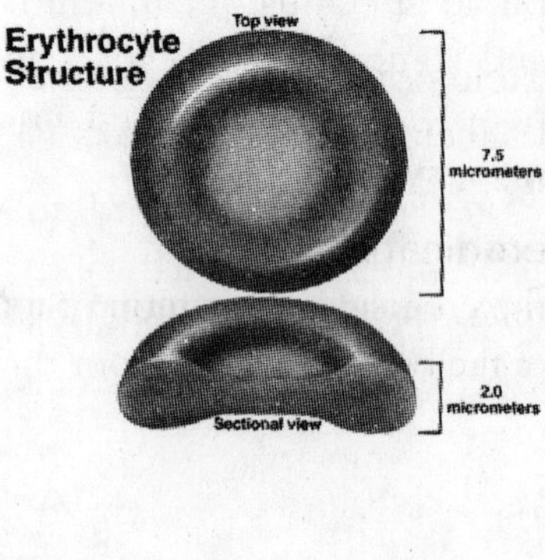

■ erythromycin
a common antibiotic used to treat bacterial infections of the skin, respiratory tract and other organs.

■ erythropoietin (epoietin, epogen)
a natural hormone that stimulates the production of red blood cells. Genetically engineered versions of EPO are used to treat anaemia due to drug toxicity. Side effects include headache and high blood pressure.

■ escape variant (escape mutant)
a drug-resistant strain, a microorganism (e.g. virus) that has mutated so as to lose its sensitivity to a drug.

■ escherichia coli
a typically harmless bacteria that is found in the human digestive tract and is present in faecal material. E. coli 0157: H7 is a pathogenic strain transmitted most commonly by undercooked meats, raw milk and person-to-person contact. This strain may cause bloody diarrhoea and can lead to haemolytic uremic syndrome, a rare but occasionally fatal kidney disorder.

■ oesophageal candidiasis
a fungal infection of the oesopha-

gus that may cause painful swallowing, leading to weight loss. Oesophageal candidiasis is an AIDS-defining opportunistic infection.

■ **esophagitis**

inflammation of the oesophagus. In some cases, this is considered an AIDS-defining condition.

■ **oesophagus (*adjective* oesophageal).**

the swallowing tube, muscular; about 9 inches long, the portion of the digestive canal between the oral cavity and the stomach.

■ **estradiol**

a potent natural form of estrogen produced by the ovaries, placenta and testes.

■ **estrogen**

a female sex hormone, a natural or synthetic substance (e.g., estradiol, Premarin) that stimulates the development of female secondary sex characteristics and regulates the reproductive cycle in women. Estrogens are known to affect the immune system.

■ **ethambutol (myambutol)**

an oral drug used in combination with other agents to treat tuberculosis and Mycobacterium avium complex (MAC) disease. Side effects may include nausea, headache, visual disturbances and joint pain.

■ **etiology**

the cause of a disease and the study of causes of disease.

■ **euthanasia**

'mercy killing', the deliberate ending of life to reduce pain and suffering.

■ **ex vivo**

outside of or removed from the body of a living organism.

■ **exacerbate**

to worsen or make more severe.

■ **exanthem (roseola)**

a rash occurring as a symptom of an acute viral disease. Exanthem subitum or roseola infantum is a common viral disease of infants and children caused by infection with human herpes virus type 6 and characterised by sudden onset of rash accompanied by fever.

■ **excision**

the process of cutting out or otherwise removing a section of tissue.

■ **exclusion criteria**

see **inclusion/exclusion criteria**

exo-

prefix, outside, the external part of the body or an organ.

■ **exocrine gland**
a gland with ducts (e.g., sebaceous glands) that deposits secretions directly to a site of action rather than into the bloodstream. Contrast with endocrine gland.

■ **exogenous**
originating or produced outside the body.

■ **exon**
an extraneous segment of genetic material (DNA) that is not expressed as proteins.

■ **exotoxin**
a toxic substance produced and released by bacteria.

■ **expanded access**
a program that makes experimental drugs available on a wide basis to patients who don't qualify for a clinical trial. In most cases, a drug with an expanded access program is already in the final stages of the approval process. The program was started in 1987 by the U.S. FDA.

■ **experimental drug**
a substance that is currently undergoing clinical trials.

■ **extracorporeal**
outside of the body.

■ **extrapolation**
the process of inferring unknown information by comparison with data that is known.

■ **extrapulmonary**
outside of the lungs.

■ **factor viii**
a protein in the blood that promotes clotting. Some haemophiliacs lack factor VIII and use a replacement derived from multiple blood/plasma donors. Many haemophiliacs were infected with HIV prior to widespread antibody testing of donated blood.

■ **failure to thrive**
a condition in which a child loses or fails to gain weight and grows at a slower rate than expected. Failure to thrive may be due to faulty metabolism, illness or malnutrition. HIV positive children often exhibit failure to thrive.

■ **fallopian tube (oviduct)**
one of the tubes leading from the ovaries to the uterus, through which an ovum (egg) travels.

■ **false-negative**
a negative test result for a person who does in fact have the disease or condition being tested for.

■ **false-positive**
a positive test result (e.g., from an HIV antibody test) for a person who does not in fact has the disease or condition being tested for. See also false-negative.

■ **famciclovir (famvir)**
an anti-herpes drug approved for the treatment of varicella-zoster virus infection.

■ **FDA**
see **Food and Drug Administration**

■ **febrile**
having fever or increased body temperature.

■ **fellatio**
oral sex on a man, sexual contact between one person's tongue and/or mouth and a man's penis and/or scrotum.

■ **fibroblast**
a cell which produces the collagen fibres that make up the connective tissue.

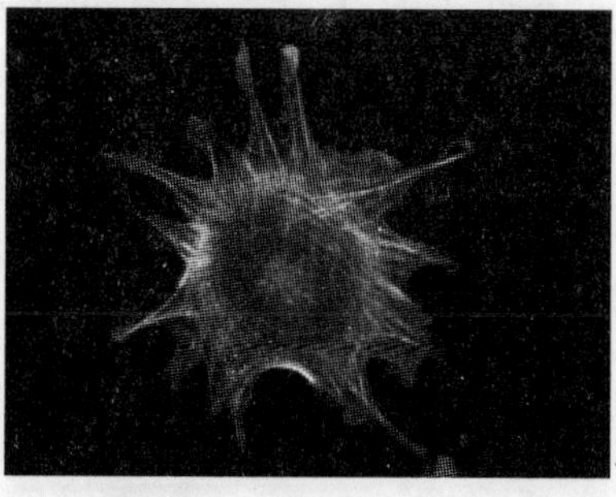

■ **first-line treatment**
the preferred standard therapy for a particular condition.

■ **fissure**
a crack or tear in the skin or a mucous membrane.

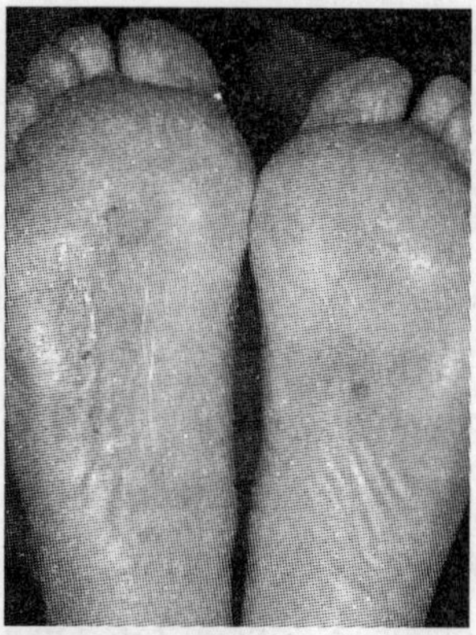

■ **flagyl**
brand name of metronidazole.

■ **floater**
a moving spot that appears in the field of vision. Floaters may be early signs of an eye disorder such as CMV retinitis.

■ **flora**
the plant and/or bacteria species that inhabit a particular environment, e.g., intestinal flora.

■ **florid**
having a bright red colour.

■ **fluconazole (diflucan)**
an anti-fungal drug used to treat fungal infections including cryp-

tococcal meningitis and oesophageal candidiasis. Side effects may include nausea, rash, abdominal pain and headache.

■ **flucytosine (5-fc, ancobon)**
an anti-fungal drug used with amphotericin B to treat cryptococcal meningitis.

■ **flush**
a sudden reddening of the skin, especially of the face and trunk.

■ **FNP**
Family Nurse Practitioner.

■ **focal**
localised, concentrated in a specific area.

■ **folate**
a vitamin necessary for red blood cell production and proper neurological function. Levels may be reduced in individuals with severe or persistent infection or those taking certain drugs. Folate is a salt or ester of folic acid.

■ **folic acid**
a B complex vitamin, important for red blood cell production. Deficiency can cause loss of taste and anaemia. Folinic acid is an active form of folic acid.

■ **follicle**
a small sac or pore. Hair follicles are depressions in the skin from which hair shafts grow. Ovarian follicles are the site of ovum (egg) production.

■ **Follicle-Stimulating Hormone (FSH)**
a hormone produced by the pituitary gland that stimulates the ovarian follicles to mature and produce ova (eggs) in women and induces sperm production in men.

■ **follicular dendritic cell**
a specialised cell in lymph nodes that traps and concentrates foreign antigens for recognition by lymphocytes.

■ **folliculitis**
an inflammation of the hair follicles which may lead to deeper abscesses. Folliculitis is often caused by bacteria (e.g., Staphylococcus aureus). Types include eosinophilic folliculitis and idiopathic folliculitis.

■ **Food And Drug Administration (FDA)**
the federal agency responsible for regulating the development, use and safety of drugs, medical devices, food, cosmetics and related products.

■ **foscarnet (foscavir)**
an antiviral drug used to treat cytomegalovirus (CMV) disease

and acyclovir-resistant herpes simplex virus and varicella-zoster virus infection. Adverse side effects include nausea, kidney toxicity and skin ulcers.

foscavir
brand name of foscarnet.

free radical
a molecule that contains at least one unpaired electron. Free radicals (reactive oxygen species) are a byproduct of normal metabolism. They are highly reactive and bind with electrons from other molecules, potentially initiating chain reactions as successive molecules lose and gain electrons. The robbing of electrons by free radicals can disrupt normal cellular processes and cause cellular damage (oxidative stress). See also antioxidant, oxidation.

Freund's adjuvant
a medium used in vaccines to maximize immune response.

ft
pharmaceutical abbreviation, make (fac, fiat, fiant).

fta-abs
fluorescent treponemal antibody test, a confirmatory blood test for the presence of Treponema pallidum, the organism that causes syphilis.

fulminant
refers to a condition that is severe or aggressive.

fundoscopy
examination of the interior of the eye with an instrument (fundoscope) that allows the examiner to peer into the eyeball through the pupil. Fundus photography is used as a diagnostic tool.

fungemia
the presence of fungi in the blood.

fungus
a plant of the subkingdom Thallophyta. A fungus lacks chlorophyll and can be a single cell or a larger plant. These are all fungus — mushroom, mould, smut, yeast. Fungi cause these diseases: candidiasis (thrush), cryptococcal meningitis, toxoplasmosis.

fusin (cxcr4, lestr)
a co-receptor on the surface of certain T-cells that, along with the CD4 molecule, allows HIV to penetrate and infect a cell.

fusion
a union or joining together into one entity.

■ G6PD
glucose-6-phosphate dehydrogenase, a human red blood cell enzyme. G6PD deficiency may cause severe anaemia. People with G6PD deficiency should not take certain medications (e.g., dapsone) due to the risk of developing anaemia.

■ gag
the gene of HIV that encodes the core proteins of the virus. Also refers to the proteins produced by the gene.

■ gamma globulin
component of blood serum (plasma) containing antibodies, sometimes abbreviated as IgG.

■ gamma interferon
see **interferon**

■ ganciclovir (DHPG, cytovene)
an antiviral drug used to treat cytomegalovirus (CMV) infection. Ganciclovir may be administered intravenously via an indwelling central catheter or via an intra-ocular implant. An oral form is used as maintenance therapy for CMV retinitis. It may also be effective for primary prophylaxis. Side effects of ganciclovir include neutropenia.

■ ganglion (plural ganglia)
a cluster of nerve tissue primarily composed of neuron cell bodies.

■ gastric
relating to the stomach.

■ gastritis
inflammation of the mucosal lining of the stomach.

■ gastroenteritis
inflammation of the mucous membrane of the stomach or intestine.

■ gastrointestinal
pertaining to the stomach and intestines.

■ gastrointestinal tract
the digestive system consisting of the mouth, stomach, small intestine, large intestine and anus.

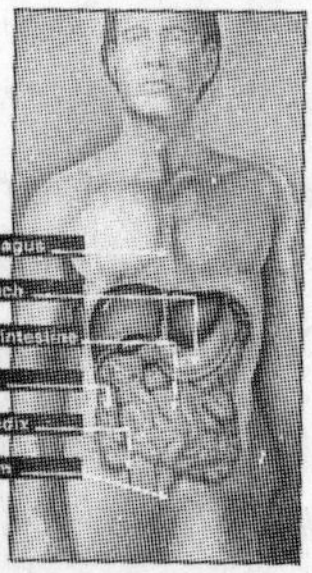

■ gay bowel syndrome
an obsolete term used to refer to a collection of enteric (intestinal) parasitic diseases commonly seen in gay men and associated with anal intercourse and/or oral-anal sexual contact.

gem 91
an experimental anti-HIV compound. GEM 91 is an antisense (complementary) strand of nucleotides that can bind to HIV RNA and block viral replication.

gene (adjective genetic)
the unit of heredity. A gene contains hereditary information encoded in the form of DNA and is located at a specific position on a chromosome in a cell's nucleus. Genes determine many aspects of anatomy and physiology by controlling the production of proteins. Each individual has a unique sequence of genes or genetic code.

gene expression
the production of a particular gene product or protein.

gene product
the protein encoded by a specific gene.

gene therapy
an approach to preventing and/or treating disease by replacing, removing or introducing genes or otherwise manipulating genetic material. Examples include adding a gene to a cell to produce a specific missing protein, using antisense molecules to prevent viral replication and altering CD4 cells to make them resistant to HIV infection. Genes may be introduced by direct injection or using a harmless viral vector to deliver genes into the cells.

generic name
a common name used to identify a drug, as opposed to a brand name used by a particular company (e.g., TMP-SMX is the generic name of the drug sold as Bactrim or Septra).

genetic engineering
manipulation of an organism's genetic material to modify the proteins it produces.

genital
refers to the reproductive or sexual organs.

genital herpes
see Herpes Simplex Virus.

Genital Ulcer Disease (GUD)
one of several, usually sexually transmitted diseases (e.g., syphilis, chancroid) that are characterised by the development of ulcers on the skin or mucous membranes. The presence of ulcers may facilitate the transmission of HIV and other STD.

genital warts
see **condylomata acuminata**

■ genito-urinary

refers to the systems and organs of reproduction and urination, especially in men where the two systems share some organs in common.

■ genome (adjective genomic)

the unique genetic code or hereditary material of an organism, carried by a set of chromosomes in the nucleus of each cell. The human genome contains an estimated 50,000-100,000 genes. The genome of HIV contains 9 genes.

■ genotype

the specific genetic makeup or 'blueprint' of an individual. Contrast with phenotype.

■ germinal centre

a part of the lymph node in which lymphocyte proliferation and maturation takes place and where T-cells are 'educated' to recognize antigens.

■ gestation

pregnancy.

■ GI

see **gastrointestinal.**

■ giardiasis

infection with a Giardia protozoan (e.g., Giardia lamblia), which is spread via contaminated food or water and by faecal-oral contact. Giardia infects the intestines and produces nausea, cramping and diarrhoea.

■ gingivitis

gum disease. Inflammation of the gingiva, which may be accompanied by pain and/or bleeding. Gingivostomatitis is a combined inflammation of the gingiva and other oral mucous membranes. See also periodontal disease.

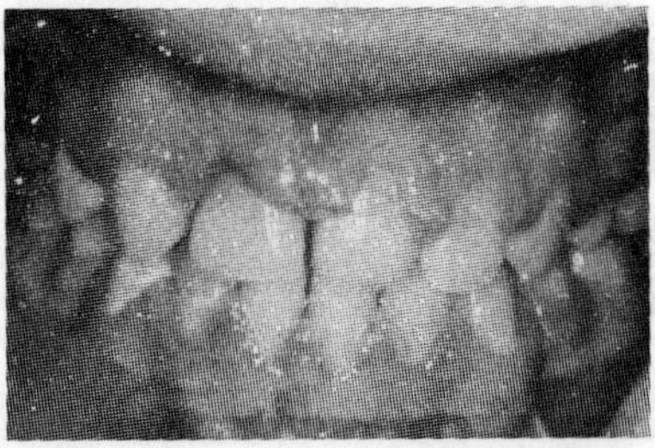

■ glaucoma

a disease of the eye marked by increased pressure within the eyeball. If left untreated, glaucoma can damage the optic nerve and cause loss of vision.

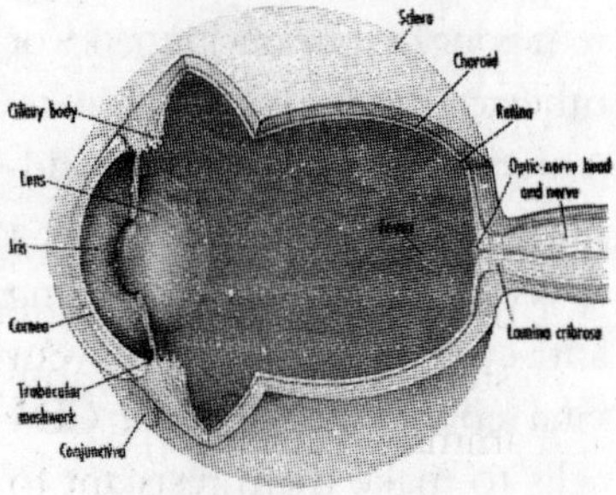

■ glial cells
non-neuronal cells that perform support functions in the brain, providing structure and assisting metabolism. AIDS dementia complex is believed to involve infection of glial and other support cells.

■ gliosis
a proliferation of glial cells in the brain. A condition frequently seen in people with HIV-related dementia.

■ globulin
a blood protein.

■ glomerulonephritis
an inflammatory disorder of the glomeruli of the kidney, often due to the build-up of immune complexes.

■ glomerulus (plural glomeruli, adjective glomerular)
one of the small units in the kidney made up of capillaries and nerve fibres where blood filtration takes place.

■ gluco-corticoid
a steroid-like substance (e.g., cortisol) capable of influencing metabolism, regulating the immune system and exerting an anti-inflammatory effect.

■ glucose (blood sugar)
a form of sugar that is the body's primary fuel; glucose broken down from food can be converted into energy or stored. Abnormally low or high levels of glucose in the blood often indicate metabolic disturbances (e.g. diabetes).

■ glutathione
an antioxidant containing the amino acid cysteine which is needed for cellular production of energy and proper immune function. Glutathione has been reported to suppress HIV in vitro and may reduce HIV-related apoptosis (cell death).

■ glycoprotein (gp)
a small unit made up of a sugar and a protein molecule, often part of a cell's membrane. Glycoproteins make up the envelope of HIV (e.g., gp120, gp160 [numbers denote molecular weight]).

■ gm
pharmaceutical abbreviation, gram.

■ GM-CSF
see Granulocyte Macrophage Colony-Stimulating Factor.

■ gonad
an organ that produces gametes (ova and sperm), i.e., an ovary or a testis.

■ **gonadotropin**
a hormone (e.g., follicle-stimulating hormone) that acts on the gonads to promote their growth and function.

■ **gonococcal**
related to infection with the Neisseria gonorrhoeae organism (e.g., gonococcal urethritis, gonococcal vaginitis).

■ **gonorrhea**
a sexually transmitted disease caused by the bacteria Neisseria gonorrhoeae. Gonorrhea may be asymptomatic or may include symptoms such as urethritis, discharge, pelvic pain and inflammation of the tissues of the genitals, rectum and/or throat. Untreated gonorrhea may spread to the upper genital tract and lead to pelvic inflammatory disease (PID) in women and may become disseminated, affecting other organs such as the heart and brain.

■ **gp120**
glycoprotein on the outer surface of HIV that binds to proteins (CD4) on helper T-lymphocyte cell (t-cell). This is HIV's docking mechanism.

■ **gp160**
a glycoprotein in the outer envelope of HIV which enables the virus to enter human cells. The glycoprotein is produced by the viral env gene and cleaved into gp120 and gp41 fragments.

■ **gp161**
HIV's recursor protein, which is split into the gp41 and gp120 surface protein by enzymes during a late stage of the replication process.

■ **gp41**
protein on the outer surface of HIV that can pierce the surface of a helper T-lymphocyte cell (T-cell) This is HIV's infection mechanism.

■ **graft**
a transplant. A tissue or organ transferred from one individual to another..

■ **Graft-Versus-Host Disease (GVHD)**
a condition in which transplanted immune tissue, e.g. bone marrow cells, attack the tissues of the new host's body.

■ **gram**
a metric unit of weight, 1 ounce is about 28 grams.

■ **gram stain**
a method used to identify bacteria by injecting a crystal violet stain

that is either lost or retained when the bacteria are rinsed, depending on the characteristics of the bacterial cell wall.

■ **gram-negative**
refers to bacteria that have a thick double cell wall that contains lipopolysaccharide or endotoxin. These bacteria lose a violet stain when rinsed.

■ **gram-positive**
refers to bacteria that have a single cell wall that does not contain lipopolysaccharide; these bacteria retain a violet stain when rinsed.

■ **granulocyte**
a type of white blood cell (basophil, eosinophil, neutrophil) that contains granules of toxic chemicals that are released to fight micro-organisms. These toxins let them digest bacteria.

■ **Granulocyte Colony-Stimulating Factor (G-CSF)**
a natural hormone that stimulates growth of granulocytes, a type of white blood cell. G-CSF manufactured by genetic engineering (Neupogen) is used to treat or prevent neutropenia associated with the use of certain drugs. Side effects include nausea, rash and bone pain.

■ **Granulocyte Macrophage Colony-Stimulating Factor**
a hormone that stimulates growth of granulocytes and macrophages. Synthetic GM-CSF (Leukine) is used to treat or prevent neutropenia caused by certain drugs. Side effects include fever, rash and bone pain.

■ **granulocytopenia**
a condition indicated by a low number of granulocytes, leading to a high risk of bacterial infection.

■ **granuloma**
an inflammatory lesion containing phagocytes.

■ **grey matter**
refers to the tissues of the brain that make up the cortex. Contrast with white matter.

■ **growth factor**
a factor responsible for regulating cell proliferation, development, migration, differentiation and/or activity.

■ **growth hormone**
see **human growth hormone**

■ **gtt**
pharmaceutical abbreviation, drop, drops (gutta, guttae).

■ **Guanine (G)**
one of the purine nucleic acid

bases that make up nucleotides, the building blocks of DNA and RNA.

■ GUD
see genital ulcer disease.

■ guillain-barré syndrome
an acute disease that produces fever and nerve inflammation resulting in bilateral weakness or paralysis, most commonly in the legs and feet.

■ gut
the intestines.

■ gynaecology
the study and treatment of the genital and reproductive system of women.

■ gynaecomastia
greater than normal breast development in males, may be a side effect of drugs that mimic female hormones.

■ h
pharmaceutical abbreviation, hour.

■ h.s.
pharmaceutical abbreviation, at bedtime (hora somni).

■ HAART
Highly Active Antiretroviral Therapy, a term for aggressive anti-HIV treatment.

■ haemophilus influenzae
a rod-shaped bacteria that occurs in the human respiratory tract and causes acute infections (e.g., pneumonia, meningitis). The bacterium was once believed to be the cause of the flu, which is now known to be caused due to a virus.

■ hairy leukoplakia
a white lesion on the cheeks, gums or tongue, possibly related to Epstein-Barr Virus infection. This is considered as an AIDS-defining condition.

■ half-life
the time required for half the amount of an agent, e.g. drug, virus, cell type to be eliminated from the body.

■ HBV
abbreviation, hepatitis B, a viral liver disease. It can be chronic or acute (life-threatening).

■ hby-097
an experimental, non-nucleoside reverse transcriptase inhibitor drug.

■ HCG
see **human chorionic gonadotropin.**

■ HCT
see **hematocrit.**

■ **helper cell (t4 cells, cd4 cells)**
a subset of T cells that carry the T4 marker and are essential for turning on antibody production, activating cytotoxic T cells and initiating other immune responses. The number of T4 cells in a blood sample is used to measure the health of the immune system in people with HIV.

■ **Helper T-Cell**
see **CD4 cell.**

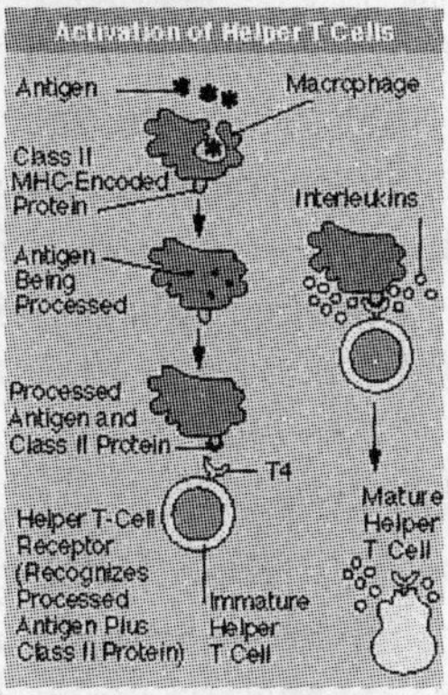

■ **helper-suppressor ratio**
see **CD4/CD8 ratio.**

■ **hematocrit (HCT)**
the percentage of red blood cells in a given amount of whole blood. The hematocrit reflects oxygen-carrying capacity. A drop in hematocrit may indicate bone marrow dysfunction. Red blood cells normally constitute about 38-54% of the whole blood in men and about 37-47% in women.

■ **haematology**
the study of blood and blood-forming tissues.

■ **haematopoiesis**
the process by which blood cells are produced in the bone marrow. Haematopoietic stem cells give rise to all types of red and white blood cells.

■ **haematotoxic**
poisonous to the blood or blood-producing bone marrow.

■ **haemo-**
prefix, blood.

■ **haemoglobin**
a protein in the red blood cells that carries oxygen and contain iron.

■ **haemoglobinemia**
the presence of free (unbound) haemoglobin in the blood plasma.

■ **haemolysis**
the breakdown or destruction of red blood cells.

■ **haemophilia**
a disorder that prevents normal blood clotting. Haemophilia is hereditary.

haemorrhage

loss of a large amount of blood from the arteries or veins. A haemorrhage may be internal or external.

HEPA (High-Efficiency Particulate Air) filter

a type of air filter that protects against airborne transmission of tuberculosis.

heparin

a chemical found in many tissues, especially the liver, that prevents blood clotting. Heparin is released by basophils and mast cells in inflammatory and allergic responses. It is used therapeutically to prevent blood coagulation.

hepatic

pertaining to the liver.

hepatitis

an inflammation of the liver that may be caused by several agents, including viruses and toxins. Hepatitis is characterised by jaundice, enlarged liver, fever, fatigue and abnormal liver function tests. Types include hepatitis A (infectious hepatitis), hepatitis B (serum hepatitis), hepatitis C, hepatitis D (delta hepatitis) and hepatitis E. A new form, hepatitis G, has recently beene characterised.

hepatitis A (infectious hepatitis)

an inflammatory viral disease of the liver with a short incubation period. Hepatitis A virus (HAV) may be transmitted by: 1. eating contaminated food 2. by foecal-oral contact 3. through household contact. Hepatitis A may be mild to severe. The symptoms include fever, nausea and jaundice.

hepatitis B (serum hepatitis)

a viral liver disease that may be acute or chronic and can be life-threatening. Symptoms include fever, headache, muscle and joint pain, malaise, nausea and jaundice. Some individuals are chronic asymptomatic carriers. Chronic hepatitis B may result in liver cirrhosis and/or cancer. The hepatitis B virus (HBV) can be transmitted by sexual contact, shared needles or contaminated blood products. Interferon-alpha is used as a treatment. A 3-dose anti-HBV vaccine is available.

hepatitis C (formerly non-a, non-b hepatitis)

a contagious viral disease that causes inflammation of the liver. A chronic carrier state occurs in some individuals and may result in life-threatening liver damage, cirrhosis and/or liver cancer.

HCV is spread via contaminated blood products or shared needles. There is no standard treatment or vaccine.

hepatitis D (formerly delta hepatitis)

a type of hepatitis that occur only in individuals who are also infected with hepatitis B.

hepatitis E (formerly enteric or epidemic hepatitis)

a type of hepatitis caused by a virus that is common in parts of Africa and Southeast Asia. The disease is usually mild and self-limiting, except in pregnant women, who may have severe cases. Hepatitis E is shed in the faeces and can be spread by the faecal/oral route.

hepatomegaly

liver enlargement.

hepatosplenomegaly

enlargement of the liver and spleen.

hepatotoxicity

being toxic to the liver.

herbology

the therapeutic use of herbs or herbal products.

Herpes Simplex Encephalitis (HSE)

inflammation of the brain caused by infection with the herpes simplex virus.

Herpes Simplex Virus (HSV-1, HSV –2)

a herpes virus that causes blisters and recurring disease. Herpes simplex virus type 1 (HSV-1) usually produces lesions on the lips or in the mouth ('cold sores' or 'fever blisters'). HSV type 2 (HSV-2) is usually sexually transmitted and lesions generally occur in the genital and/or anal area. Blisters typically appear 2-12 days after infection and may be painful. In healthy individuals, lesions usually resolve without treatment in 2-3 weeks; in immunocompromised persons, lesions last longer, may be more frequent and severe and the virus may become disseminated. Symptomatic disease outbreaks occur at unpredictable intervals. Between outbreaks HSV lies dormant in the nerves; reactivation may result from emotional stress, physical trauma, hormonal changes or other illnesses. Outbreaks may be preceded by a numb or tingling sensation and flu-like symptoms known as the prodrome. Both HSV-1 and HSV-2 are treated with acyclovir. Ganciclovir or foscarnet are used to treat acyclovir-resistant HSV.

■ **Herpes Simplex Virus I**
the virus that causes cold sores and fever blisters.

■ **Herpes Simplex Virus II**
the virus, abbreviated HSV II, that causes genital herpes, painful lesions on the anus or genitals. HSV II can be dormant in nerve tissue but is reactivated by stress and other factors. HSV II is spread by contact with a lesion.

■ **Herpes Zoster ('shingles')**
a viral condition characterised by painful blisters that typically appear in a dermatomal (linear) distribution on the skin following nerve pathways. Blisters generally dry and scab leaving minor scarring. Shingles is caused by reactivation of a previous infection with the varicella-zoster virus (VZV) that initially causes chickenpox. VZV lies dormant in the nerves and reactivates when immune defences are weakened. Shingles outbreaks may recur more frequently and VZV may become disseminated in people with HIV disease. Disseminated herpes zoster resembles chicken pox, with a rash, fever and possibly pneumonia. Herpes zoster may also lead to ocular and neurological complications.

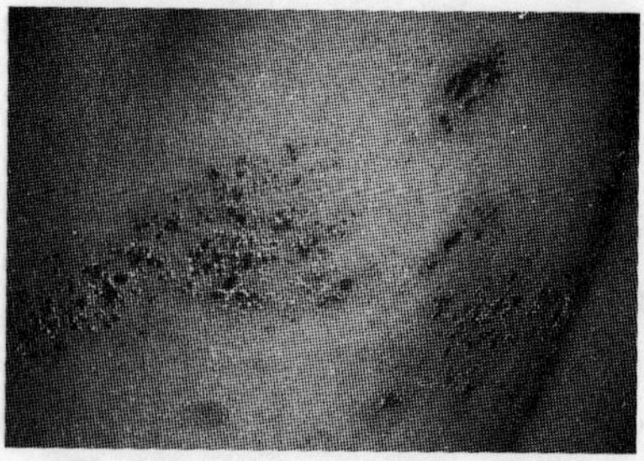

■ **Herpes virus (herpetoviridae)**
a group of viruses that includes herpes simplex virus type 1 (HSV-1 or HHV-1) and 2 (HSV-2 or HHV-2), varicella-zoster virus (VZV or HHV-3), Epstein-Barr virus (EBV or HHV-4), cytomegalovirus (CMV or HHV-5), human herpes virus types 6 and 7 (HHV-6, HHV-7) and Kaposi's sarcoma-associated herpes virus (KSHV or HHV-8). Herpes viruses may act as opportunistic pathogens and/or cofactors in HIV pathogenesis.

■ **HERS**
HIV Epidemiology Research Study.

■ **heterogeneous**
mixed, made up of diverse, dissimilar elements or parts.

■ **heterozygote (adjective heterozygous)**
an individual who possesses two different alleles or gene

variants, at a given site on a chromosome. Contrast with homozygote.

■ **hickman catheter**
a flexible tube surgically inserted into a blood vessel for infusions of medicine and nutrition over a long period of time.

■ **hirsutism**
excessive growth of bodily and facial hair in a male pattern.

■ **histamine**
a white crystalline compound involved in immune responses (hormone or chemical transmitter). It regulates the production of stomach acid and is the main cause of allergic reactions.

■ **histo-**
prefix, body tissue.

■ **histocompatibility**
immunologic identity or similarity. Histocompatibility testing compares the HLA (also called MHC) 'self' antigen markers of a tissue donor and recipient to determine whether a transplant is possible. A close match implies that the donor and recipient share the same MHC genes, reducing the chance that the transplant will be rejected.

■ **histology**
the study or examination of tissue.

■ **histopathology**
the study or examination of abnormal or diseased tissue.

■ **histoplasmosis**
a fungal infection (Hostoplasma copsulatum) that is usually confined to the Mississippi River Valley. It can cause inflammation in multiple organs, like lungs, meninges, heart, etc.

■ **historical control**
the medical records of an individual used to compare current patients receiving an experimental treatment with a similar-seeming patient treated in the past.

■ **HIV**
abbreviation, Human Immunodeficiency Virus. (see **human immunodeficiency virus**).

■ **HIV associated minor cognitive/motor disorder**
an early stage of AIDS dementia complex.

■ **HIV burden**
see **viral load.**

■ **HIV disease**
a viral infection caused by the human immunodeficiency virus.

HIV negative
showing no evidence of infection with HIV (e.g., absence of antibodies against HIV) on a blood or tissue test. See seronegative.

HIV positive
showing evidence of infection with HIV (e.g., presence of antibodies against HIV) on a test of blood or tissue. See seropositive.

HIV-associated dementia
see AIDS dementia complex.

hives
itchy, raised, swollen areas on the skin or mucous membranes, often a manifestation of an allergic reaction. (*syn.,* urticaria).

hivid
brand name of ddC.

HIVIG
concentrated anti-HIV immunoglobulins used in passive immunotherapy. HIVIG is under study, as a treatment for children with HIV disease and as a therapy to prevent vertical transmission. Side effects include headache, fever and rash.

HLA
abbreviation, see **human leukocyte antigen**

Hodgkin's disease
a progressive cancer of the lymphatic system, characterised by the presence of Reed-Sternberg cells, enlarged lymph nodes and spleen, wasting, fever and anaemia. The disease is treated with chemotherapy and radiation.

holistic
an alternative treatment system that focuses on the whole person rather than on specific diseases or disorders and considers physical, emotional, social, environmental and spiritual factors.

homeopathy
a treatment methodology based on the theory that 'like cures like'. Homeopathic therapy uses extremely small, diluted doses of substances that normally cause the types of symptoms one is seeking to treat.

homeostasis
maintenance of equilibrium or a stable bodily state, e.g. body temperature, fluid composition.

homology
similarity or correspondence. Homologous DNA is similar at matched positions, e.g. SIV and HIV-2 are 70% homologous. Homologous blood or tissue

transfers are transfers or transplants from one individual to another. Contrast with autologous. (*adjective* homologous).

■ **homozygote**
an individual who possesses 2 copies of the same allele or gene variant, at a given site on a chromosome. Contrast with heterozygote. (*adjective* homozygous).

■ **hormone**
a substance created by one organ, transmitted to another organ by the blood, that causes some activity in the second organ due to a chemical reaction. For example, testosterone is a hormone found only in males.

■ **Hormone Replacement Therapy (HRT)**
the administration of exogenous hormones (typically estrogen) to replace those that the body is not able to produce (e.g. due to menopause or hysterectomy). HRT is used to relieve symptoms of hormonal deficiency (e.g. hot flashes, osteoporosis).

■ **host**
a cell or organism within which a parasitic organism lives.

■ **hpmpc**
see **cidofovir.**

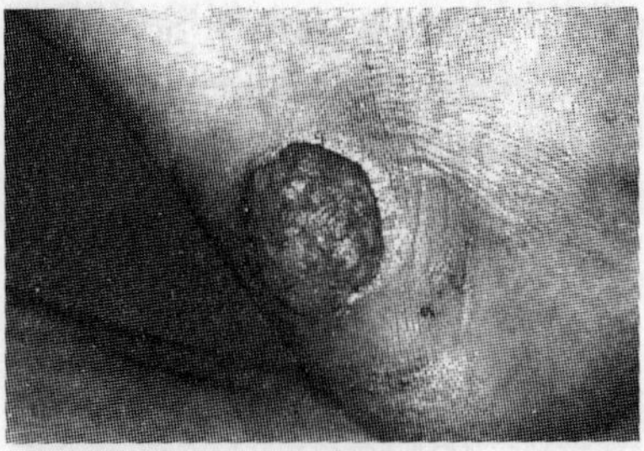

■ **HSV**
herpes simplex virus.

■ **HTLV-i/HTLV-ii**
see human T-cell leukemia virus.

■ **HTLV-III**
one of the original names given to the virus now known as HIV.

■ **Human Chorionic Gonadotropin (HCG)**
a hormone secreted by the placenta that maintains pregnancy during the early development of the embryo. HCG is made up of 2 subunits, alpha and beta. The beta subunit (bHCG) has been shown to suppress the development of Kaposi's sarcoma cells in vitro.

■ **Human Growth Hormone (HGH)**
a peptide hormone secreted by the anterior pituitary gland. HGH enhances growth by stimulating metabolism and protein synthesis and also stimulates the immune system. Recombinant hu-

man growth hormone (Serostim) is a genetically engineered drug used for the treatment of HIV-related wasting syndrome. Side effects include muscle pain, oedema and carpal tunnel syndrome.

■ human herpes virus 6

herpes virus that infects lymphocytes, including CD4 cells. HHV-6 infection generally occurs early in life and may cause fever, exanthem (roseola, a red skin rash) in infants. HHV-6 is associated with neuropathology, chronic fatigue syndrome, multiple sclerosis and certain autoimmune diseases.

■ human herpesvirus 7

herpesvirus that infects human T-cells, but is not known to cause disease. (hhv-7).

■ human immunodeficiency virus

a slow-acting retrovirus of the lentivirus family, believed to be the sole or primary cause of AIDS. HIV is transmitted sexually, through blood or vertically (from mother to child). There are 2 known types: HIV-1 and HIV-2.

■ human immunodeficiency virus (type I)

the cause of HIV Disease and AIDS, a retrovirus (lentivirus family) that attacks the immune system. Formerly called HTLV III and LAV.

■ human immunodeficiency virus (type II)

a retrovirus closely related to simian immunodeficiency virus (SIV) and less closely related to HIV-1. HIV-2 is found primarily in West Africa. Symptoms of HIV-2 infection are similar to those of HIV-1 but are typically milder and take longer to develop. There are 5 known types of HIV-2 (A through E).

■ human leukocyte antigen

a genetic marker of 'self' which prevents the immune system from attacking the body's own tissues. Various HLA patterns are associated with (HLA).

■ hyper-

prefix, over, above, beyond, excessive.

■ hypersensitivity

an overreaction, especially as a reaction to a drug.

■ hypo-

prefix, below, under, less than normal.

■ iatrogenic

refers to an unfavourable response to medical or surgical treatment; symptoms attributable to a medical therapy (e.g., peripheral neuropathy caused by an antiviral drug). See also nosocomial.

■ **ic**

abbreviation, see **inhibitory concentration.**

■ **id**

pharmaceutical abbreviation, intradermal.

■ **idiopathic**

refers to a disease or condition of unknown cause or origin.

■ **Idiopathic Cd4 T Lymphocytopenia (ICL)**

immunosuppression and low CD4 cell count with no detectable cause. ICL syndrome has been called 'non-HIV AIDS'.

■ **idiotype**

the unique part of the variable region of an antibody. The idiotype can in turn act as an antigen for other antibodies (anti-idiotypes).

■ **IDU**

injection drug user, especially illegal drugs.

■ **IDVU**

intravenous drug user, especially illegal drugs.

■ **ig**

immunoglobulin. See **antibody.**

■ **igg**

gamma globulin. Component of blood serum (plasma) containing antibodies.

■ **il**

pharmaceutical abbreviation, intralesional.

■ **im**

pharmaceutical abbreviation, intramuscular.

■ **immune**

exempt, not affected, not responsive.

■ **immune based therapy**

see **immunotherapy**.

■ **immune complex**

a cluster formed when an antigen and an antibody (or multiple antigens and antibodies) bind together. Immune complexes may circulate in the blood or lodge in tissues, where they can lead to physiological damage.

■ **immune modulating therapy**

see **immunotherapy.**

■ **immune modulator**

see **immunomodulator.**

■ **immune response**

the activity of the immune system, (e.g., against a micro-organism or cancerous cell).

■ **immune restoration**
rebuilding of a damaged or compromised immune system i.e. immune reconstitution.

■ **immune surveillance**
the immune system's recognition of and defence against foreign organisms and cancerous cells.

■ **immune system**
the body's defence system that protects against foreign invaders (e.g., micro-organisms) and cancerous cells. Some immune defences are non-specific (e.g., phagocytosis). Defences against specific antigens are of 2 types: cell-mediated (TH1) and humoral (antibody-based or TH2). Organs of the immune system include the lymph nodes, spleen, thymus, tonsils and bone marrow.

■ **Immune Thrombocytopenic Purpura (ITP)**
an immune disorder that results in a low number of platelets in the blood. A common disorder in people with HIV, it often resolves as immune deficiency worsens. HIV-related ITP usually does not have serious consequences. Its cause has not been definitely determined, but probably has to do with the large number of antibody-antigen complexes sponged up by platelets. Antibody-coated platelets are destroyed in the spleen. Treatment with AZT (Zidovudine) or an Intravenous Immunoglobulin (IVIG) frequently alleviates the condition.

■ **immunity**
natural or acquired resistance to a specific disease.

■ **immunisation**
the process by which a person is protected against the adverse effects of infection by a disease-causing micro-organism. Active immunisation (vaccination) involves inoculating a person with an antigen and relying on their body to mount an immune response. Passive immunisation involves giving the patient exogenous (manufactured or transferred from another individual) antibodies.

■ **immunise**
to render immune.

■ **immuno-**
prefix, immunity.

■ **immunocompetent**
capable of mounting an appropriate immune response.

immunocompromise
reduction in immune system function.

immunodeficiency
the inability of the immune system to work properly, resulting in susceptibility to disease. Immunodeficiency may be either congenital (present from birth) or acquired. HIV leads to immunodeficiency by attacking T-cells.

immuno-endocrinology
a hybrid branch of medicine that combines the study of the immune system (immunology) and the study of the endocrine glands and their hormones (endocrinology).

immunofluorescence assay
a test that uses a glowing dye to identify pathogenic organisms.

immunogen
an antigenic agent that stimulates an immune response.

immunogenic
producing immunity.

immunogenicity
the ability to stimulate an immune response.

immunoglobulin
one of a group of blood serum proteins that can act as an antibody.

immunoglobulin A (IGA)
a type of antibody found in body fluids and the mucous membranes lining the openings of the body. IgA is the basis of mucosal immunity, attacking pathogens at the site of entry into the body.

immunoglobulin D (IgD)
a specialised immunoglobulin of unknown function, found in small amounts in the serum.

immunoglobulin E (IgE)
a type of antibody associated with mast cells. IgE is responsible for immediate hypersensitivity (allergic) reactions and immune defence against parasites.

immunoglobulin G (IgG, gamma globulin)
the most common type of antibody in the plasma. IgG provides specific immunity against particular antigens and is a major defence against bacteria, viruses and toxins. IgG initiates the complement cascade that result in the destruction of the membrane of pathogens. IgG extracted from donor plasma (gamma globulin) is used for passive immunisation.

immunoglobulin M (IgM)
a type of antibody that (along with IgG) provides specific hu-

moral immunity against bacteria and viruses.

immunology (adjective immunologic)

the study and/or treatment of disorders that involve the immune system (e.g., cancer, HIV disease, autoimmune diseases).

immunomodulator (immune)

an agent or process capable of modifying or influencing the function of the immune system. Immune modulators include cytokines (e.g., IL-2, gamma interferon) and broad-acting agents.

immunostimulant (immunopotentiator)

an agent that stimulates or enhances the function of the immune system.

immunosuppression

reduced function of the immune system; a state in which the immune system defences have been suppressed, damaged or weakened.

immunotherapy (immune-based therapy)

a therapy that attempts to modify or enhance immune response or reconstitute a damaged immune system. Examples of immune-based therapies for HIV disease include active immunisation (vaccination), passive hyperimmune therapy, CD8 cell line expansion and cytokine therapy.

impairment

dysfunction, damage or deterioration.

in

(*pharmaceutical abbreviation*), intranasal.

in situ

occurring in place or at a specific site. Carcinoma in situ is a tumour that has not invaded surrounding tissues.

in situ hybridisation

a method used to detect and locate specific DNA or RNA sequences.

in utero

in the uterus. Typically refers to events that occur in the womb before birth.

in vitro

in an artificial environment, especially test tube experiments involving a reaction of human tissue. [*Latin* - in glass]

in vivo

within a living organism, especially lab experiments. [*Latin* - in a living body]

■ inactivate

to eliminate the activity or effectiveness of an agent or substance.

■ incidence (incidence rate)

the number of new cases of a diseases or condition in a specific population over a given period of time. The incidence rate is determined by dividing the number of new cases by the total population.

■ inclusion/exclusion criteria

characteristics of an individual which qualify or disqualify them from taking part in a clinical trial (e.g., CD4 cell count, pregnancy, other drugs taken).

■ incontinence

loss of voluntary control over urination and/or defecation.

■ incubation period

the time between an initial exposure to an infectious agent and the development of symptoms of disease.

■ IND

(*pharmaceutical abbreviation*), investigational new drug.

■ indication

purpose of a drug.

■ indinavir (crixivan, formerly mk-639)

a protease inhibitor drug approved for the treatment of late-stage HIV disease. Current practice favours the use of indinavir in combination therapy (e.g., with nucleoside analog drugs) to avoid the development of drug-resistant virus.

■ induction

the initiation phase of a particular therapy.

■ induration

a swelling and hardening of soft tissue caused by infiltration of macrophages and CD4 cells. Injection of a substance (e.g., tuberculin PPD) and 'reading' of the resulting induration is used to detect previous exposure to an organism or to gauge the strength of the immune response.

■ inert

inactive; having no biological or catalytic activity.

■ infection

a condition in which the body is invaded by an infectious organism (e.g., bacterium, virus, fungus). An active infection is one that leads to disease symptoms, while a latent infection remains dormant within the body.

infectious
capable of being transmitted from one individual to another, for example through sexual contact.

infertility
diminished or absent ability to conceive. Infertility may due to a variety of causes, including abnormal hormonal levels, low sperm production and scarring of the fallopian tubes.

infiltration
the process of passing through tissues or through a semi-permeable medium or filter.

inflammation
the body's response to tissue injury or infection, which typically includes increased vessel dilation and permeability, resulting in redness, swelling, heat and pain.

Inflammatory Bowel Disease (IBD)
a disorder of the colon that causes stomach pain, constipation and diarrhoea.

influenza
the flu; an infectious respiratory disease contracted by inhaling a virus. Influenza is characterised by chills, fever, prostration, headache, muscle aches, sore throat and a dry cough. Influenza may be life-threatening in infants, the elderly and persons with compromised immune systems.

informed consent
a way to protect people entering a drug trial. Each participant in a clinical trial must sign a consent form that explains the purpose of the trial, the results expected, the mechanics of the trial, potential risks, a list of other treatments that are available. There is also a statement telling the participant that one can leave the clinical trial at any time.

infusion
the introduction of a solution into a vein, especially medicine or nutritional supplements.

inguinal
relating to the groin.

inhibitor
a substance used to retard or stop an undesirable reaction.

Inhibitory Concentration (IC)
a measure of the efficacy of a drug. The IC50 is the concentration of a drug that eliminates 50% of a population of microorganisms.

Injection Drug User (IDU)
a person who uses a drug (e.g.,

heroin, cocaine) that is administered with a needle and syringe. The term intravenous drug user (IVDU) is also sometimes used. IDU is more general and refers to injection methods other than intravenous administration.

■ **inoculation**
the introduction of a pathogen or antigen into the body, especially to stimulate antibody production or other immune responses.

■ **inpatient**
a patient who is treated in a hospital or other medical facility.

■ **insomnia**
inability to sleep.

■ **institutional review board**
a committee, commonly abbreviated IRB, at an institution or hospital involved in biomedical research that oversees all human trials.

■ **Institutional Review Board (IRB)**
a committee of physicians, medical experts, researchers and community members which is responsible for ensuring that clinical trials conducted by a hospital or other institution are safe and ethical.

■ **insulin**
a peptide hormone produced by the Islets of Langerhans cells in the pancreas. Insulin enables the body to metabolise and use glucose. Lack of or insensitivity to insulin results in diabetes.

■ **Insulin-Like Growth Factor (IGF)**
a substance naturally produced by the body that has many of the same effects as growth hormone. There are 2 types, IGF-1 and IGF-2, a genetically engineered form of IGF-1 is under study as a therapy for AIDS-related wasting.

■ **integrase**
a viral enzyme that enables the integration of viral genetic material into a host cell's DNA.

■ **integrase inhibitor**
an antiviral drug (e.g., zintevir) that blocks viral replication by interfering with the action of the integrase enzyme.

■ **integration**
the process by which viral DNA is integrated into or made part of, the genetic material of a host cell. Viruses integrate their genetic material into a host cell and 'take over' its biological mechanisms to self-replicate.

intent-to-treat

a method of analysis in clinical trials that groups each participant according to the arm to which they were initially assigned, e.g., experimental drug, standard therapy, placebo, regardless of whether they remain in that arm for the duration of the study.

interaction

a change in the way one drug acts when it is taken with some other drug or substance. Also called drug interaction.

Intercompany Collaboration For Aids Drug Development

a cooperative effort of several large pharmaceutical companies to share drugs and data and to collaborate on trials of experimental HIV/AIDS drug combinations.

interferon

a protein in a cell produced to prevent replication of a virus in the cell.

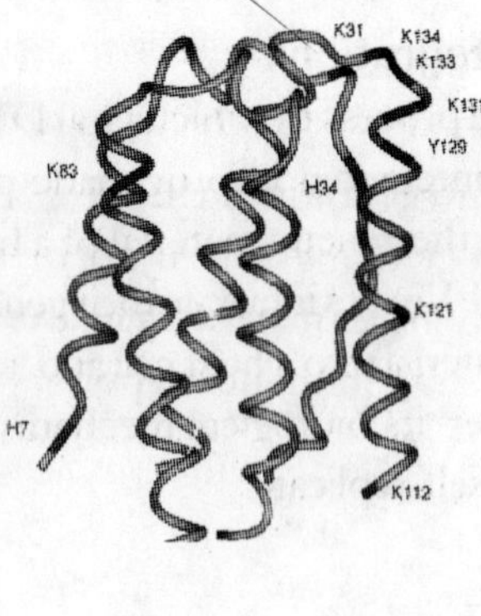

interferon-alpha (intron-a, roferon-a)

a type of interferon produced in response to viral infection. Genetically engineered interferon-alpha is used to treat Kaposi's sarcoma, ano-genital warts and hepatitis B and C and is under study as an anti-HIV therapy. Side effects include flu-like symptoms, anaemia and neutropenia. A low-dose oral formulation of interferon-alpha (Kemron) has shown little efficacy.

interferon-beta

a type of interferon that typically has less severe side effects than interferon-alpha. Interferon-beta is used to treat multiple sclerosis and is under study as a treatment for human papillomavirus (HPV) infection.

interferon-gamma (immune interferon, actimmune)

a type of interferon produced by CD8 and CD4 cells. Interferon-gamma is used to treat leprosy and is under study as a treatment for toxoplasmosis, PCP and MAC.

Interleukin

a hormone (cytokine) that acts as a messenger in the immune system.

■ **Interleukin (IL)**

a cytokine (chemical messenger) secreted by immune system cells that regulates a range of immune system functions. Types include IL-1, IL-2 (T-cell growth factor), IL-10 and IL-12.

■ **Interleukin 1 (IL-1)**

a cytokine released by monocytes, macrophages and other immune cells that fight infection. IL-1 activates helper T-cells, mediates acute systemic immune symptoms (e.g., fever) and acts on the hypothalamus to decrease appetite.

■ **Interleukin 10 (IL-10)**

a cytokine released by TH2 T-cells that stimulates the proliferation and activity of B-cells, modulates macrophage function and enhances humoral (TH2) immunity, while suppressing cell-mediated immune function.

■ **Interleukin 12 (IL-12)**

a cytokine produced by lymphocytes (e.g., monocytes, macrophages, dendritic cells, neutrophils) that activates natural killer cells and cytotoxic T-lymphocytes and induces the production of interferon-gamma. IL-12 is associated with the cell-mediated (TH1) immune response. Recombinant IL-12 is under study as a immunomodulatory treatment for HIV disease.

■ **Interleukin 2 (IL-2, I-cell growth factor)**

a cytokine produced by activated CD4, cells that promotes the proliferation and activity of CD4 cells, CTL and natural killer cells. IL-2 is associated with cell-mediated (TH1) immune response. Recombinant IL-2 (Aldesleukin, Proleukin) is used for cancer therapy and is under study as a immunomodulatory treatment for Kaposi's sarcoma and HIV disease. Side effects include flu-like symptoms (fever, chills), decreased blood pressure and anorexia.

■ **Interleukin 3 (IL-3)**

a haematopoietic factor that promotes the growth and differentiation of several types of blood cells (red, white and platelets).

■ **Interleukin 4 (IL-4)**

a cytokine released by the TH2 subset of CD4 cells that stimulates antibody production.

■ **Interleukin 6 (IL-6)**

a cytokine produced by macrophages that mediates acute systemic immune responses (e.g., fever).

■ **intermittent**
occurring sporadically or in phases.

■ **interstitial**
refers to the spaces between cells.

■ **intolerance**
inability of the body to appropriately metabolise an agent or drug, often characterised by adverse side effects.
intra-
prefix, within.

■ **intra-**
prefix, within, internal.

■ **intracellular**
within a cell.

■ **intracranial**
within the skull.

■ **intracutaneous**
within the skin.

■ **intraepithelial neoplasia**
abnormal cell growth that suggests possible malignancy. Common sites are the anus (anal intraepithelial neoplasia) and the uterine cervix (cervical intraepithelial neoplasia).

■ **intralesional**
within a lesion, especially an injection.

■ **Intramuscular (IM)**
administered into a muscle.

■ **intraocular**
administered into the eye. An intraocular implant is embedded in the eye and releases a drug slowly over time.

■ **intrapartum**
during child birth.

■ **intrathecal**
injected into the fluid (theca) around the spinal cord.

■ **intrauterine**
within the uterus.

■ **Intrauterine Device (IUD)**
a contraceptive device, typically made of plastic and sometimes including copper, that is placed within the uterus to prevent pregnancy.

■ **intravaginal**
introduced into the vagina.

■ **intravenous**
within a vein, especially a drug injection.

■ **Intravenous (IV)**
injected directly into a vein.

■ **Intravenous Immune Globulin (IVIG)**
broad-spectrum concentrated antibodies administered intravenously to treat conditions in which the body does not produce enough of its own antibodies. Recombinant and pooled

immunoglobulins from blood donors are used to prevent bacterial infections, especially in children with HIV disease.

■ **intravitreal**

within the eye.

■ **invasive**

refers to a procedure that involves entry into or invasion of the body (e.g. making an incision, inserting an instrument). Also refers to a cancer that spreads from its original site to other parts of the body.

■ **invasive cervical cancer**

an aggressive type of cancer of the uterine cervix that has spread beyond the surface cell layers. Invasive cervical cancer is more common and spreads more rapidly in women with HIV disease and is an AIDS-defining illness.

■ **Investigational New Drug (IND)**

an FDA classification applied to experimental drugs undergoing trials to assess safety and efficacy prior to marketing approval in U.S.. IND status must be granted before a drug can enter Phase I testing.

■ **involution**

atrophy, shrinkage or loss of normal shape and structure.

■ **IRB**

Institutional Review Board. A committee at an institution or hospital involved in biomedical research that oversees all human trials.

■ **iron**

an important trace element needed for the production of red blood cells. Iron deficiency can lead to anaemia.

■ **irrigate**

to wash out or rinse with a fluid.

■ **iscador**

extract of the European mistletoe plant under study as a immunomodulatory therapy.

■ **Islets Of Langerhans (islet cells)**

cells in the pancreas that produce insulin.

■ **isolate**

a specific individual microbe and its genetically identical progeny.

■ **isoniazid (INH)**

an antibiotic used in combination regimens to treat tuberculosis. Side effects include liver toxicity and peripheral neuropathy.

■ **itraconazole**

a triazole antifungal drug used to treat various fungal diseases (e.g., cryptococcosis, histoplasmosis).

Side effects include nausea and headache.

■ iu

pharmaceutical abbreviation, international unit.

■ International Unit (IU)

a standardised unit of measurement.

■ IUD

see **Intrauterine Device**.

■ IVIG

see **intravenous immune globulin.**

■ jaundice

yellow discoloration of the skin and whites of the eyes, caused by the inability of the liver to break down the pigment bilirubin. Jaundice is often associated with liver damage or disease, e.g. hepatitis, with gallbladder disease and with the excessive destruction of red blood cells.

■ JC Virus

see **Progressive Multifocal Leukoencephalopathy**

■ Kaposi's Sarcoma (KS)

an abnormal or cancerous proliferation of cells and blood and/or lymph vessels, causing tumours on the skin, mucous membranes and/or internal organs. KS typically appears as pink or purple flat or raised lesions. Types include classic KS, African KS and AIDS-related or transplant-related KS. KS is associated with a herpes virus (KSHV or HHV-8). It occurs more commonly among HIV positive gay and bisexual men than among others with HIV disease, indicating that it may be sexually transmitted.

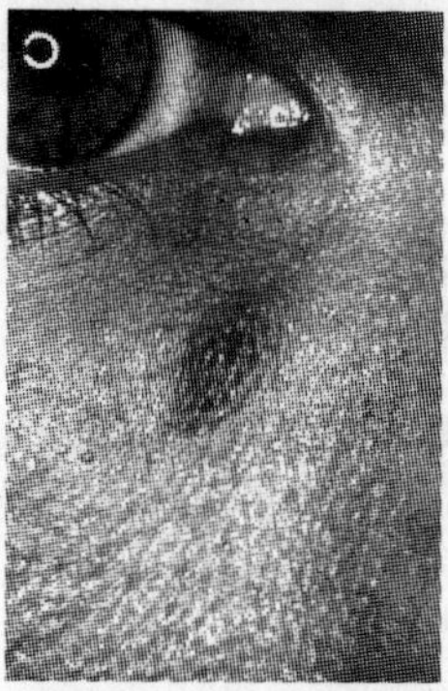

■ Kaposi's Sarcoma-Associated Herpes Virus (KSHV)

a recently discovered herpes virus found in samples of tissue from Kaposi's sarcoma lesions and believed to be a causal agent or co-factor.

■ Karnofsky Score

a subjective score (0-100) given by a doctor to describe a patient's ability to perform everyday tasks (eating, dressing, etc.).

■ keratitis

inflammation of the cornea of the eye.

■ **keratosis**

a skin condition characterised by overgrowth and thickening of the outer skin layers. A skin lesion marked by flat or elevated growth. Keratosis may develop into squamous cell carcinoma. Types include actinic keratosis and seborrheic keratosis.

■ **ketoconazole (nizoral)**

an imidazole drug used to treat systemic fungal or yeast infections (e.g., candidiasis, histoplasmosis). Side effects include liver toxicity.

■ **ketotifen**

an antihistamine drug that lowers TNF-alpha levels and is under study as an immunomodulatory therapy for HIV disease.

■ **kg**

kilogram, a measure of weight equal to 2.2046 pounds.

■ **kidney (adjective renal)**

one of the 2 bean-shaped organs located in the lower back part of the abdominal cavity. The kidneys filter out the waste material from the blood and excrete it as urine.

■ **kidney stone (nephrolithiasis)**

an accumulation, e.g. of calcium in the kidney, which may lead to pain and blockage.

■ **killer cell**

a lymphocyte that can kill cancerous and virus-infected cells. Killer cells are neither T-cells nor B-cells, but belong to a third class of lymphocytes.

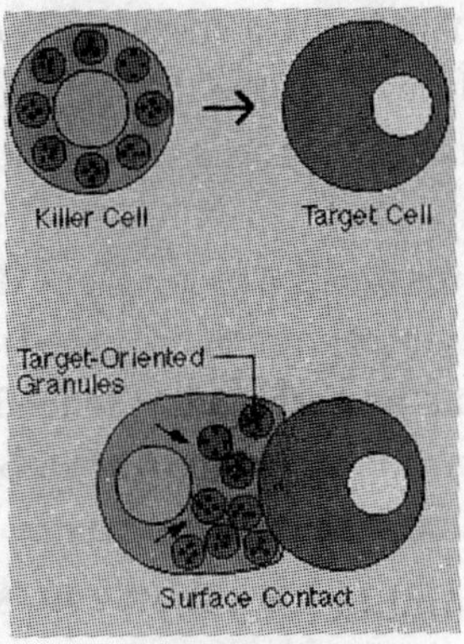

■ **killer T cells**

an immune system cell (cytotoxic lymphocyte) that directly kills other infected cells in the body (e.g., cancer cells, cells infected by a virus). Also called natural killer cells.

■ **killer t-cell**

see cytotoxic T-lymphocyte.

■ **kinase**

an enzyme that adds phosphates to amino acids, a crucial step in intracellular signalling and many other processes.

■ **klebsiella**

a type of bacteria that can cause respiratory disease (e.g., sinusitis, pneumonia), especially in immunocompromised individuals.

■ Koch's Postulates

a method for determining whether a specific micro-organism causes a specific disease. The micro-organism must be seen in all cases of the disease, isolated and grown in a laboratory, the laboratory-grown micro-organisms must cause the same disease when administered to a test animal and the same type of micro-organism must then be isolated from the animal.

■ kombucha

a colony of yeast organisms, sometimes referred to as a 'mushroom', that is grown in water or tea to produce a fermented drink which is claimed to have natural antibiotic and immune-enhancing properties.

■ kupffer cell

a type of specialised macrophage in the liver.

■ L drug

a group of experimental non-nucleoside reverse transcriptase inhibitor drugs.

■ labia

lips or the rounded folds of skin that surround the vaginal and urethral openings in the female.

■ lactation

milk production.

■ lactobaccilus acidophilus

bacteria that make up part of the normal flora of the human intestine, mouth and vagina. Some types of yogurt contain acidophilus and may help restore normal bacterial balance.

■ lak cell

see **lymphokine-activated killer cell**.

■ lamivudine

see **3TC**

■ langerhans cell

a type of dendritic cell in the skin and mucous membranes that transports antigens to the lymph nodes.

■ laparoscopy

a procedure in which a small, lighted instrument is inserted through an abdominal incision for the purpose of diagnosis, biopsy or surgery.

■ Large Simple Trial (LST)

a trial that includes a large number (typically several thousand) people and extends over a long period of time. LST has a broad eligibility criteria, simple enrolment procedures, collect minimal data and use major illness or death as endpoints. LST are intended to study treatments under 'real world' conditions of use.

■ latency (adjective latent)
the state in which a pathogenic organism is present in the body but not actively replicating or causing illness, i.e. being present but not evident. In HIV Disease, the virus is present for years before any symptoms appear. During this period of latency, the virus is still active and damaging the immune system.

■ lateral
pertaining to the side (as opposed to the midline) of the body.

■ late-stage disease
advanced progression of a disease. Late-stage HIV disease occurs 5-10 or more years after initial HIV infection and is characterised by low CD4 cell counts, high viral load levels, wasting syndrome and possibly the presence of multiple opportunistic infection symptoms.

■ LAV
see **lymphadenopathy-associated virus.**

■ lavage
the washing out of an organ or cavity, for example to obtain a sample for diagnosis.

■ LD
see **lethal dose**

■ Lean Body Mass
muscle and organ tissue.

■ LEEP
see **Loop Electrocautery Excision Procedure**

■ legionellosis (legionnaire's disease)
an upper-respiratory tract infection caused by Legionella bacteria, which are widely distributed in nature and may be spread via contaminated water supplies. Infection is often acquired nosocomially (in a hospital).

■ leishmaniasis
an infection caused by the protozoan parasite Leishmania that infects and lives inside human macrophages. The parasite is transmitted by sandflies. The infection is characterised by lesions on exposed parts of the body and may be fatal if left untreated.

■ lentinan
an extract from the shiitake mushroom that has been used in Japan as an adjunct to cancer therapy. Lentinan may stimulate immune functions such as natu-

ral killer cell activity and cytokine production.

■ lentivirus

a subfamily of retroviruses that includes HIV. Lentiviruses kill cells and are associated with chronic, slow-developing diseases.

■ leprosy

a disease caused by Mycobacterium leprae, characterised by skin lesions and necrosis. There are 2 forms of leprosy, lepromatous and tuberculoid.

■ lesion

a wound or injury.

■ lethal dose (ld)

a measure of the lethality or toxicity of an agent. The LD50 is the amount of a micro-organism or a substance which will kill 50% of the subjects to which it is administered.

■ leucovorin

a derivative of folic acid, a member of the vitamin B complex. Leucovorin protects cells from the cyto-toxic effects of certain drugs (e.g., dapsone, trimetrexate) and is used to prevent drug-induced anaemia.

■ leukemia

a group of diseases involving an abnormal production of white blood cells.

leuko-, leuk-, leuco-, leuc-
prefix, white.

■ leukocyte

white (actually colourless) blood cell.

■ leukocytosis

abnormally high number of white blood cells.

■ leukopenia

abnormally low number of white blood cells.

■ leukoplakia

see **oral hairy leukoplakia.**

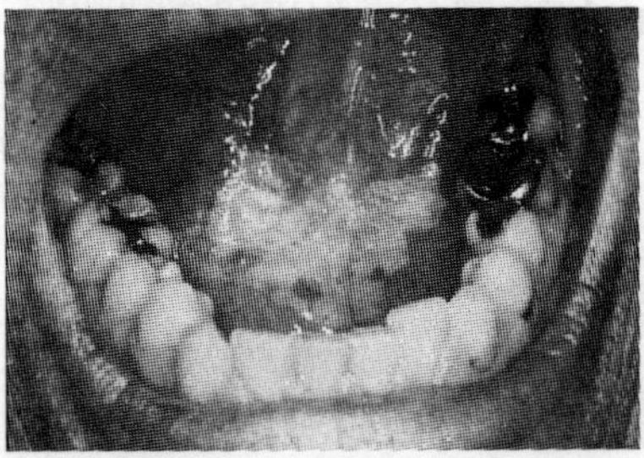

■ leukopoiesis

formation and development of white blood cells.

■ leukotriene

a chemical compound in leukocytes that mediates allergic and inflammatory reactions.

■ levofloxacin

a broad-spectrum quinolone antibiotic used to treat respiratory infections.

■ **LIP**
Lymphocytic Interstitial Pneumonia.

■ **lipid**
a fat.

■ **lipogenesis**
production of lipids (fats).

■ **Lipopolysaccharide (LPS)**
a molecule composed of fat and sugar. LPS is produced by certain bacteria and makes up part of their cell wall. When the bacteria die, the toxin is released, leading to the release of cytokines resulting in symptoms of chills, fever and possibly shock.

■ **lipoprotein**
a compound composed of protein and fats.

■ **liposomal daunorubicin (dox-sl)**
a liposomal form of daunorubicin used to treat Kaposi's sarcoma.

■ **liposome (lipid vesicle)**
a spherical fat particle suspended in a liquid. Liposomes are used to carry drugs or other substances to cells or tissues, allowing them to remain active longer in the body and have a less detrimental effect on the liver.

■ **listeriosis**
a serious, sometimes fatal, bacterial disease [Listeria (L.monocytogenes)] that looks like severe encephalitis but with paralysis. This is considered as an AIDS-defining condition.

■ **live-attenuated virus**
an altered live used in vaccines to provoke an immune response. Live-attenuated vaccines may induce longer-lasting protection that whole-killed virus, but involves some risk of back-mutation to the original, more virulent wild-type.

■ **liver (adjective hepatic)**
a large organ in the upper abdominal cavity that cleanses toxins and dead cells from the blood and is important in metabolic transformation of various substances. The liver is responsible for excreting drugs and alcohol from the body and many drugs can be toxic to the liver.

■ **liver enzyme**
a protein produced by the liver (e.g. SGOT, SGPT) that catalyses various physiological reactions. Abnormally high levels of liver enzymes in the blood may indicate liver damage or disease.

■ **Liver Function Test (LFT)**
a blood test that measures levels of liver enzymes to indicate how

well the liver is working and whether it might be inflamed or damaged.

■ localised

affecting a specific bodily site organ or system. Contrast with systemic.

■ locus (plural loci)

a place or site.

■ log

a measure based on the logarithmic scale that refers to quantities in factors of 10. A log change is an exponential or 10-fold increase or decrease (e.g., 10 to 100 is a 1-log increase, 1,000,000 to 10,000 is a 2-log decrease.) Changes in viral load are often expressed in logs.

■ Long Terminal Repeat (LTR)

a segment of the HIV gene that must be activated to 'turn on' viral replication.

■ longitudinal

refers to a study that follows participants over an extended period of time.

■ Long-Term Nonprogressor (LTNP)

an individual who has been infected with HIV for several years (7-10 or more) but does not exhibit immune system decline or has opportunistic diseases. About 10% of persons with HIV disease seem to be LTNP. LTNP typically has a strong cytotoxic T-lymphocyte response, minimal lymph node damage and a relatively low viral load. LTNP may have unusually strong immune responses, may be infected with a weakened strain of HIV or may have protective genetic factors.

■ Long-Term Survivor (LTS)

an individual who has been infected with HIV for several years (typically 7-10 or more years). The term long-term survivor may include both long-term nonprogressors and individuals who live for many years with a damaged immune system and/ or opportunistic infections.

■ Loop Electrosurgical Excision Procedure (LEEP)

use of a heated wire loop to remove a cone-shaped wedge from the bottom of the uterine cervix for biopsy. The procedure is similar to a cone biopsy, but is generally faster and heals more rapidly.

■ loperamide (imodium ad)
an anti-diarrhoea drug.

■ low-dose oral interferon-alpha (kemron)
a form of the cytokine interferon-alpha that is administered in low doses under the tongue.

■ LTR
see **Long Terminal Repeat.**

■ LTR Inhibitor
a substance that interferes with the long terminal repeat of the HIV gene, thus inhibiting viral replication.

■ lumbar puncture (spinal tap)
the insertion of a needle into the subarachnoid space of the spinal column to remove cerebrospinal fluid for diagnosis or to inject medications or anaesthesia.

■ lupus
see **systemic lupus erythematosus.**

■ Luteinising Hormone (LH)
a hormone that stimulates the maturation and release of ova (eggs) in females and the production of testosterone by Leydig cells of the testes in males.

■ lymph
a clear or yellowish fluid containing white blood cells and some red blood cells that travels through the lymphatic system. The lymph system helps remove bacteria and some proteins from tissues. It also transports fat to the intestines.

■ lymph node (lymph gland)
a small, bean-sised organ located throughout the body, with concentrations in the neck, groin and armpits. Lymph nodes filter out antigens and are the site of antigen presentation and immune activation. They supply lymphocytes to the blood stream and remove bacteria from the body. The lymph nodes are a reservoir site for HIV.

■ lymphadenopathy
inflammation (swelling) of lymph nodes caused by numerous conditions, including flu, mononucleosis, lymphoma and primary HIV infection.

■ Lymphadenopathy-Associated Virus (LAV)
an early name for the virus, now known as HIV.

■ lymphatic system (adjective lymphoid)
a network of capillary-like vessels, ducts, nodes and organs that help maintain the fluid environ-

ment of the body and coordinate immune responses. Two major lymphatic vessels return fluid to the vascular system. The lymphoid organs include the lymph nodes, spleen, thymus, tonsils and adenoids.

- **lymphoblastosis**
  the production of lymphocytes.

- **lymphocyte**
  a T-cell or B-cell, white blood cells responsible for immune defence.

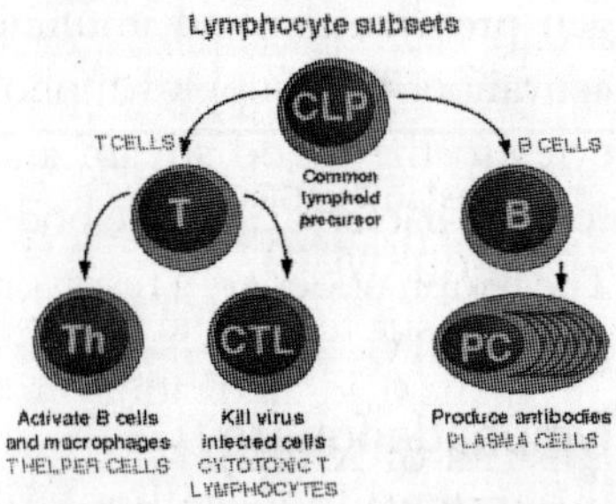

- **lymphocytic interstitial pneumonia**
  a kind of pneumonia common in children with HIV Disease.

- **lymphocytopenia**
  reduced numbers of white blood cells (e.g., CD4 cells).

- **Lymphoid Interstitial Pneumonia (LIP)**
  a rare type of pneumonia that particularly affects children with AIDS.

- **lymphokine**
  a chemical messenger (e.g., interferon, interleukin) produced by lymphocytes that directs and regulates immune responses by stimulating macrophages, killer cells and other lymphocytes.

- **Lymphokine-Activated Killer cell (LAK cell)**
  a type of lymphocyte (neither a T-cell nor a B-cell) that has cytotoxic activity against a broad range of cells and is not MHC-restricted.

- **lymphoma**
  cancer of the lymphatic system

- **lymphopenia**
  a decreased number or proportion of lymphocytes in the blood.

- **lymphoproliferative**
  refers to the proliferation or replication of lymphocytes.

- **lysis**
  rupture and destruction. May refer to rupture of a cell or to the breakdown of a molecule or compound (e.g., hydrolysis).

- **m.**
  pharmaceutical abbreviation month

- **m.ft.**
  pharmaceutical abbreviation, mix and make (miscre et fiat)

m.t.
(*pharmaceutical abbreviation*), send like this (mitte talis)

mac
abbreviation, mycobacterium avium complex a disease caused by a dust particles. Symptoms include weight loss, fatigue and fever. MAC is considered as an AIDS-defining condition.

macro-
prefix, large.

macrolide
one of a group of antibiotic drugs (e.g., clarithromycin, azithromycin) related to erythromycin.

macrophage
a large (phagocytic) cell in the immune (reticuloendothelial) system. This is the reconnaisance unit of the blood stream, circulating, looking for foreign matter, alerting (by producing neopterin) the entire immune system if there is a problem.

MACS
see **Multicentre AIDS Cohort Study**

macula
the pigmented central area on the retina that is devoid of blood vessels. The macula is the most sensitive area of the retina and is responsible for retinal nourishment. Macular degeneration refers to the atrophy of the macula, which may lead to vision loss.

maculopapular eruption
a rash with both flat and raised lesions or sores.

magnesium (mg)
a mineral necessary for proper metabolism. Magnesium deficiency may worsen sensory neuropathy and affect immune function.

Magnetic Resonance Imaging (MRI)
a diagnostic technique that uses magnetic fields and radio waves (instead of X-rays). MRIs produce a 3 dimensional computer model.

MAI
see **Mycobacterium avium complex.**

mainstream treatment/therapy
use of drugs that are standard therapy for a given condition, typically drugs that have been approved by the FDA and are prescribed by doctors for the specific indication. Contrast with alternative therapy.

■ maintenance therapy (secondary prophylaxis)
preventive therapy that follows successful initial treatment of an illness. Generally, maintenance therapy continues for the lifetime of the patient to prevent disease recurrence.

■ Major Histocompatibility Complex (MHC)
a group of genes that control the expression of cell surface protein markers (also known as human leukocyte antigen or HLA markers) that determine receptor shape and allow immune cells to recognize components of the body (i.e., to distinguish 'self' from 'non-self'). MHC molecules are necessary for antigen presentation and for recognition of antigens by immune system cells. Each individual has one of a variety of genetically determined MHC/HLA patterns. There are two classes of MHC molecules, MHC-I and MHC-II.

■ mal-
prefix, bad, abnormal.

■ malabsorption
ineffective or substandard absorption of nutrients or drugs in the intestines.

■ malaise
a generalised feeling of illness and discomfort.

■ malaria therapy (Induced Malaria Therapy, IMT)
a proposed therapy for HIV disease in which a patient is infected with a malaria-causing parasite in the hope that the ensuing immune response and high fever will kill HIV.

■ malignancy
a tumour, cancer or an abnormal growth that tends to metastasize (spread).

■ malignant
refers to a cancer, neoplasm or tumour that grows in an uncontrolled manner, invading nearby tissue and spreading (metastasizing) to other sites through the bloodstream. Contrast with benign.

■ malnutrition (malnourishment)
lack of the minimum amount of fluids, proteins, carbohydrates, lipids, vitamins, minerals and other nutrients essential for sound health and growth. Faulty nutrition may result from poor diet, lack of appetite or abnormal absorption of nutrients from the gastrointestinal tract.

■ mantoux test
see **PPD test.**

■ marijuana
see **cannabis.**

■ marinol
brand name of dronabinol.

■ marker
a lab result or symptom observation used to measure a treatment's effectiveness or an individual's immune system status. Also refers to a unique identifier on a cell's surface.

■ marrow
the soft tissue filling a cavity in bones, consisting of fat cells and maturing blood cells.

■ marrow suppression
a side-effect of some drugs that leads to a decrease in white blood cells, red blood cells and platelets.

■ mast cell
a basophil (a type of granular white blood cell) that has left the bloodstream and entered a tissue. Mast cells release histamine and heparin, chemicals which mediate allergic reactions.

■ maternal-foetal transmission
see **vertical transmission.**

■ maximum tolerated dose
the largest dose of a drug a patient can take without unacceptable adverse side effects.

■ MBACOD
a chemotherapeutic cancer treatment regimen that combines the drugs methotrexate, bleomycin, doxorubicin (Adriamycin), cyclophosphamide, vincristine (Oncovin) and dexamethasone.

■ mcg
microgram.

■ MDR-TB
see **Multidrug-Resistant Tuberculosis.**

■ measles
an acute contagious viral disease marked by an eruption of distinct red circular spots on the skin.

■ meatus
an opening or channel through a part of the body or from the body to the outside, e.g. the urinary meatus.

■ megadose
a far greater than normal dose, especially of vitamins.

■ megakaryocyte (thromboblast)
a large, multilobed cell in the bone marrow that gives rise to platelets.

■ **megestrol acetate**
a synthetic progesterone used to stimulate appetite and promote weight gain in people with HIV-related wasting syndrome. Side effects may include menstrual changes in women, feminising side effects in men and swelling of the hands and feet.

■ **melanoma**
a cancer derived from melanin-producing cells.

■ **membrane**
a thin sheet or layer of pliable tissue serving as a semi-permeable covering.

■ **memory cell**
a cell that remains after the body mounts an immune response to an antigen and is capable of an immediate response to the reappearance of the same antigen. Memory cells include certain subsets of T-cells (CD4 and CD8) and some B-cells.

■ **memory T-cell**
blood cells (T-cells) that have a receptor for a specific antigen that was previously encountered by the immune system. These cells proliferate, providing a quick response to pathogens.

■ **meningismus**
stiffness of the neck resulting from infection and/or inflammation of the membranes covering the brain and spinal cord.

■ **meningitis**
inflammation of meninges, usually a bacterial infection.

■ **meningoencephalitis**
inflamation of the brain or meninges.

■ **meninx (pl. meninges)**
a membrane that encloses the brain and spinal cord.

■ **menopause**
the cessation of menstruation. Menopause may be due to hormonal changes, surgery or drug use. Natural menopause typically occurs between 45 and 60 years of age; women with HIV may experience early menopause.

■ **menstruation (menses)**
a stage of the female reproductive cycle. An ovum (egg) matures and is released every month. Hormones are released to prepare the uterus for possible implantation. If pregnancy does not occur, the uterine lining (blood and tissue) is shed and expelled (the menstrual period).

■ **messenger RNA**
pieces of ribonucleic acid that carry genetic information from

DNA to ribosomes, leading to the synthesis of new proteins.

■ **metabolism**

the process of building the body's molecular structures from nutrients (anabolism) and breaking them down for energy production (catabolism).

■ **metastasis**

secondary cancer that has spread from the primary or original site to another part of the body.

■ **methadone**

an oral opioid drug used for pain therapy and to treat opiate (e.g., heroin) addiction. Methadone maintenance therapy is used to prevent withdrawal symptoms by administering a small dose of methadone on a regular, e.g. daily basis.

■ **methamphetamine**

a drug that exerts a stimulatory effect on the nervous system.

■ **methemoglobin**

a form of haemoglobin that is unable to combine reversibly with and thus transport, oxygen.

■ **metronidazole**

an antibiotic drug used to treat giardiasis and under study for the treatment of microsporidiosis.

■ **micro-**

prefix, small.

■ **microbe**

a tiny living organism (e.g., bacterium, protozoan, fungus), especially those which cause disease.

■ **microbicide**

an agent that inactivates, kills or destroys microbes.

■ **microcephaly**

a birth defect characterised by an abnormally small head, incomplete development of the brain and usually mental retardation.

■ **microglia**

cells within the brain that are related to macrophages.

■ **microgram (mcg)**

a unit of weight equivalent to one-millionth of a gram (10-6g). 1,000 micrograms equals 1 milligram.

■ **micron**

a micrometre or one-millionth of a metre.

■ **micronutrient**

a trace element; an organic compound small amounts of which are essential for physical health, growth and metabolism.

■ **microorganism**

a tiny organism (e.g., bacterium).

■ **microscopy**
examination using a microscope, a magnifying instrument.

■ **microsporidiosis**
infection (Microsporidia protozoal pathogen) that causes diarrhoea and cramps. This is sometimes incorrectly diagnosed as cryptosporidiosis.

■ **milligram (mg)**
a unit of measurement, 1,000 milligrams equal 1 gram.

■ **mineral**
a carbonless inorganic element that promotes enzymatic reactions within the body and is necessary for proper cellular metabolism. Essential minerals include sodium, potassium, calcium, phosphorous and magnesium.

■ **MIP-1-alpha, MIP-1-beta**
2 chemokine proteins that affect HIV activity. MIP-1-alpha and MIP-1-beta are believed to act in conjunction with RANTES, another chemokine.

■ **mitogen**
a substance that stimulates the division of cells and can induce cancerous growth.

■ **molluscum contagiosum**
an infectious skin disease caused by a virus. Symptoms are small, white tumours on the face or body.

■ **monilia**
a group of yeast-like fungi related to Candida.

■ **mono-**
prefix, one, alone.

■ **Monoamine Oxidase Inhibitor (MAO Inhibitor)**
an older class of therapeutic drugs used to treat clinical depression.

■ **monoclonal antibodies**
artificial antibody, created in a lab and targeting a specific disease (epitope).

■ **Monoclonal Antibodies (MAB)**
antibodies derived (often by genetic engineering) from a single cell or its clones. MAB are specifically directed against a particular antigen (e.g., anti-cytomegalovirus antibodies) and are used as tools to detect and identify specific proteins.

■ **monocyte**
a large white blood cell that plays a role in immune defence, by acting as a scavenger that destroys invading micro-organisms. Monocytes circulate in the

bloodstream. When they migrate to the tissues, they mature into macrophages. Monocytes are a reservoir of HIV.

■ **monokine**
a cytokine produced by monocytes and macrophages.

■ **monomucleosis**
a disease characterised by an abnormally large number of leucocytes with single nuclei.

■ **mononeuritis multiplex**
a type of neuropathy characterised by inflammation of or damage to several nerves in unrelated parts of the body, leading to asymmetric areas of movement and sensory disorder. The condition tends to occur during the early stages of HIV infection.

■ **mononuclear cell**
a cell that has 1 nucleus, used to refer to a subset of white blood cells (e.g., lymphocytes, monocytes). Mononuclear cells may circulate in the blood (peripheral blood mononuclear cells) or reside in the lymph nodes or other tissues.

■ **mononuclear pleocytosis**
an abnormally high number of mononuclear cells.

■ **mononucleosis (kissing disease)**
an infectious disease caused by the Epstein-Barr virus that is easily transmitted via saliva. The disease is characterised by a sore throat, fatigue and possibly swollen glands or a swollen spleen.

■ **monotherapy**
use of a single drug or other therapy.

■ **morbidity**
sickness; the state of being affected by disease.

■ **morphine**
a narcotic analgesic derived from opium that has effects on the central nervous system and the bowel. Morphine is used for the relief of acute or chronic severe pain.

■ **mortality**
death. The mortality rate is the rate of death in a given population.

■ **mosaic**
a combination of different genetic variants occurring in a single individual.

■ **motility**
the ability to move.

■ **motor function**
movement functions of the body.

moxibustion

the burning of the herb moxa (mugwort) near the body, often used in conjunction with acupuncture as an element of Traditional Chinese Medicine.

MRI

Magnetic Resonance Imaging, a diagnostic technique that using magnetic fields and radio waves instead of X-rays. MRI produces a 3 dimensional computer model.

mucocutaneous

denoting the junction where mucous membrane and skin meet at the oral, vaginal and anal orifices of the body.

mucoris

infection with a Mucorales fungus. The disease may involve the brain or sinuses. Infection is rare and usually occurs in immunocompromised people.

mucosal immunity

immunity that involves IgA antibodies located in the mucous membranes at the openings of the body (e.g., the genital tract). This type of immune defence repels invaders at their point of entry.

mucous membrane (mucosa)

a moist layer of semi-permeable tissue lining the openings of the body, e.g., the gastrointestinal, respiratory and genitourinary tracts.

mucus

a thick, viscous fluid (e.g. mucin) secreted by mucous membranes that consists primarily of glycoproteins. Mucin acts as a protective barrier and lubricant.

Multicentre Aids Cohort Studies (MACS)

a set of longitudinal studies of over 5,000 gay and bisexual men in 4 U.S. cities. Long-ranging data are available for men in this cohort from as far back as 1984.

Multidrug Resistant Tuberculosis (MDR-TB)

a strain of Mycobacterium tuberculosis that is resistant to a number of the standard anti-TB drugs. Treatment requires aggressive therapy with up to 7 different drugs taken concurrently.

multinucleated

refers to a cell with more than one nucleus.

Multinucleated Giant Cell (MGC)

a cell that forms clusters in the brain. MGC are associated with HIV infection.

■ **Multiple Sclerosis (MS)**
a disease characterised by hardened plaques on the brain and spinal cord. MS can cause paralysis, tremors and speech and vision disturbances. It typically occurs in early adulthood and is characterised by exacerbations and remissions. MS has been associated with human herpes virus-6 (HHV-6) infection.

■ **multivariate analysis**
a statistical analysis technique in which multiple variables are analysed separately to determine the contribution made by each variable to an observed result.

■ **multivitamin**
a nutritional supplement that contains a variety of essential vitamins and minerals.

■ **murine**
relating to mice.

■ **musculoskeletal**
relating to the muscles and the skeletal system.

■ **mutagenicity**
ability to cause genetic mutations.

■ **mutant strain**
a new isolate produced by a change in the character of a gene.

■ **mutation**
a change in the character of a gene that is perpetuated in subsequent cell divisions.

■ **MX**
medical abbreviation for maintenance therapy.

■ **myalgia**
muscular pain

■ **myambutol**
brand name of ethambutol.

■ **myasthenia**
abnormal muscular weakness.

■ **mycelex**
brand name of clotrimazole.

■ **myco-, myc-**
prefix, fungus.

■ **mycobacteria**
a category of gram-positive, acid-fast bacteria that contains species that cause diseases such as tuberculosis, leprosy and Mycobacterium avium complex.

■ **mycobacterium**
a slender, rod-shaped bacteria of the genus Mycobacterium, including the bacteria that cause MAC and TB.

■ **Mycobacterium Avium Complex (MAC)**
a disease caused by Mycobacterium avium or Mycobacterium intracellulare (sometimes referred to as Mycobacterium avium-

intracellulare or MAI), bacteria found in soil and water. In immuno-suppressed persons, the bacteria can infect the lymph nodes, intestines, bone marrow, liver, spleen, spinal fluid, lungs and the gastrointestinal tract. MAC is the most common bacterial infection in persons with advanced AIDS (usually under 50-75 CD4 cells/ mm3). Symptoms include diarrhoea, wasting, fever, night sweats, fatigue and spleen enlargement. Clarithromycin is used as treatment and prophylaxis for MAC.

■ **mycobacterium kansasii**

an atypical mycobacterial species that usually does not cause disease in humans, but may do so in immuno-compromised individuals.

■ **mycobacterium tuberculosis**

commonly called tuberculosis or TB, a bacterial infection.

■ **mycoplasma**

a micro-organism, of which there are many varieties, e.g. Mycoplasma penetrans, that usually does not cause disease in people with healthy immune systems. Mycoplasma is believed by some to be a co-factor in the development of AIDS.

■ **mycosis**

1. a fungal growth in the body.
2. a disease caused by fungus (e.g., candidiasis, cryptococcosis, histoplasmosis).

■ **mydriatic**

a drug that produces dilation of the pupils.

■ **myelin**

a white fatty substance that forms the sheath around the axons of some neurons and provides insulation necessary for proper neural transmission.

■ **myelo-, myel-**

prefix, spinal cord, marrow.

■ **myelocyte**

a type of immature white blood cell, normally found in the bone marrow.

■ **myeloma**

a malignant tumour of the bone marrow.

■ **myelopathy**

a disease or disorder of the bone marrow.

■ **myelosuppression**

inhibition of bone marrow activity, causing decreased production of blood cells.

■ **myelotoxic**
destructive to the bone marrow.

■ **myocardium (adjective myocardial)**
the muscle layers of the heart.

■ **myoclonus**
violent, uncontrollable contractions of the muscles, either localised or occurring throughout the body.

■ **myopathy**
an inflammation or disease of the muscles that may cause pain or weakness.

■ **myositis**
inflammation of the skeletal muscle, which may involve muscle degeneration and weakness. Polymyositis simultaneously involves several muscles. Dermatomyositis is a condition characterised by both skin and muscle inflammation.

■ **n.r. (non rep.)**
pharmaceutical abbreviation, do not repeat (non repetatur)

■ **nac**
n-acetylcysteine, a substance which is converted within the body to cysteine, an amino acid that is a component of glutathione, a major cellular antioxidant. NAC may block the action of tumour necrosis factor.

■ **naive T-cell**
a subset of CD4 and CD8 cells that proliferate rapidly when exposed to new antigens. Naive cells are 'uncommitted' and respond to general antigenic stimulation i.e. not only to a specific antigen. A naive T-cell is not yet programmed to stimulate either a cell-mediated (TH1) or a humoral (TH2) response.

■ **naltrexone**
a drug used to treat opiate addiction and alcoholism. Naltrexone blocks the opiate receptors, preventing cells from responding to opiate drugs and endorphins. Naltrexone has been used as an immune modulator with some people with HIV disease.

■ **NASBA**
see **Nucleic Acid Sequence-Based amplification.**

■ **natal**
relating to birth.

■ **National Institute Of Allergy And Infectious Disease**
a component of the National Institutes of Health that conducts federally-funded research aimed at preventing, diagnosing and treating infectious dis-

eases such as AIDS and tuberculosis. NIAID conducts the majority of HIV/AIDS research in the U.S., including the AIDS Clinical Trials Group (ACTG), Community Programs for Clinical Research on AIDS (CPCRA) and the AIDS Vaccine Evaluation Group (AVEG).

■ National Institutes Of Health (NIH)

a large biomedical research organisation that is part of the U.S. Public Health Service (PHS). NIH includes various institutes, centres and divisions, several of which (e.g., NIAID) perform AIDS-related research.

■ National Science Foundation (NSF)

the agency of the U.S. federal government that coordinates and funds scientific and technological research, including medical research.

■ National Task Force On AIDS Drug Development

a task force of the Department of Health and Human Services commissioned by the president to study obstacles to AIDS drug development and formulate ways to overcome them.

■ Natural Killer Cell (NK Cell)

a type of lymphocyte that attacks and kills tumour cells and cells infected with micro-organisms. Unlike cytotoxic T-lymphocytes, NK cells are non-specific and attack infected cells without regard to specific antigens or MHC receptor configuration.

■ naturopathy

A alternative system of natural healing that relies on healthy foods and exercise and the avoidance of drugs, believing that the body can cure itself.

■ NCI

see National Cancer Institute.

■ nebuliser

a device used to convert liquid medication to a fine mist that can be inhaled.

■ necrosis

localised tissue death.

■ NEF

a gene of HIV that influences viral replication; also the protein produced by that gene.

■ nelfinavir (viracept, formerly ag1343)

a protease inhibitor drug currently in clinical trials.

■ **neo-**
prefix, new, recent.

■ **neonate (adjective neonatal)**
a newborn, especially within the first weeks after birth.

■ **neoplasia**
abnormal cell growth that may be precancerous.

■ **neoplasm**
abnormal new growth in plant or animal tissue, a tumour.

■ **neopterin**
a substance produced by macrophage cells when they find a foreign substance in the blood stream. Neopterin alerts other cells to take action against the intruder. Measuring neopterin is one way of finding out how well the immune system is working.

■ **nephro-, neph-**
prefix, kidney.

■ **nephrolithiasis**
see **kidney stone.**

■ **nephrotoxicity**
the property of being poisonous to the kidneys. Many drugs have nephrotoxic side effects.

■ **nerve**
a cordlike structure composed of fibres that conduct impulses between the central nervous system and other part of the body. A nerve cell is a neuron or cell that conducts neural impulses.

■ **Nerve Growth Factor (NGF)**
one of a family of proteins that nourish and sustain neurons.

■ **neural**
relating to a neuron, a nerve or the nervous system.

■ **neuralgia**
pain along a nerve pathway.

■ **neuritis**
inflammation of the nerves, typically accompanied by symptoms of pain and tenderness.

neuro-,neur-
prefix, pertaining to the central nervous system (brain, spinal cord)

■ **neuroimaging**
examination of the brain by external methods, e.g., magnetic resonance imaging, CT scan.

■ **neuroleptic**
a drug that acts on the nervous system and modifies psychotic behaviour.

■ **neurologic**
pertaining to the central nervous system (brain and spinal cord) or the peripheral nervous system (the nerves in the rest of the body).

neurology
the branch of medicine concerned with the nervous system and its disorders.

neuron (nerve cell)
a cell which conducts electric neural impulses from one part of the body to another. Neurons are made up of dendrites i.e. branch-like fibres receiving impulses and axons i.e. fibres which transmit impulses and communicate with other neurons and effector organs at junctures called synapses.

neuropathy
any disease, inflammation or abnormality of a nerve.

neuropathy (adjective neuropathic)
damage to the nerves. An inflammatory or degenerative condition of the nervous system.

neuropharmacologic
relating to drugs that affect the nervous system.

neuropsychological
relating to both physical and psychological aspects of the brain.

neuroradiology (neuroradiography)
the study or diagnosis of parts of the nervous system using X-rays.

neurosyphilis
a late form of syphilis that affects the brain and may lead to dementia and death.

neurotoxicity
the quality of being destructive of or poisonous to the tissues of the nervous system.

neurotransmitter
a chemical messenger, e.g., dopamine, serotonin used to communicate among neurons and between neurons and other types of cells.

neutralization
a process whereby antibodies bind to an antigen, e.g. HIV to prevent infectious or toxic processes.

neutralising antibody
an antibody that neutralises (renders harmless) infectious micro-organisms. Neutralising antibodies to HIV block the ability of the virus to infect cells. Contrast with enhancing antibody.

neutropenia
a low number of neutrophils in the blood.

neutrophil
a white blood cell (granulocytes) that is filled with chemicals that can destroy (digest) micro-organ-

isms. These cells are the body's front line defence against bacterial infection.

■ **nevirapine (viramune, formerly birg-587)**
a non-nucleoside reverse transcriptase inhibitor drug approved for the treatment of HIV disease. Nevirapine blocks HIV replication by binding to the reverse transcriptase enzyme. Side effects include rash and liver toxicity.

■ **nf-kappa b (nf-kb)**
nuclear factor kappa B, a regulatory protein that functions to increase cellular metabolic activity and cell division. Certain HIV genes contain receptors for NF-kB, which may induce increased HIV gene expression and thus viral replication.

■ **NHL**
abbreviation, non-Hodgkin's lymphoma, a rare cancer that affects B-cells in the lymph system.

■ **niacin**
a vitamin needed for the metabolism of proteins, carbohydrates and fats. Signs of niacin deficiency include weakness, headache, skin rash and diarrhoea.

■ **NIAID**
see **National Institute of Allergy and Infectious Disease.**

■ **night sweats**
abnormal sweating during sleep.

■ **NIH**
see **National Institutes of Health.**

■ **nitric oxide**
a reactive oxygen intermediate (free radical) that has several biological functions.

■ **nitrite inhalant (poppers)**
a volatile (easily evaporated) chemical preparation with vasodilating (blood vessel expanding) properties. Some forms (e.g., amyl nitrite, isobutyl nitrite or Rush) may be used recreationally to enhance sexual sensation. Some studies have linked inhalant use to immunosuppression and they were previously regarded by some as a cofactor for AIDS and/or Kaposi's sarcoma.

■ **NNRTI**
see **Non-Nucleoside Reverse-Transcriptase Inhibitor.**

■ **nociception**
the perception of pain or injury. A nociceptor is a pain receptor.

■ **nodule**
a hard, raised area of the skin or a mucous membrane, a knot or swelling.

nongonoccocal cervicitis
inflammation of the uterine cervix caused by an organism other than Neisseria gonorrhoeae, e.g. Chlamydia trachomatis, Trichomonas vaginalis.

Nongonoccocal Urethritis (NGU)
inflammation of the urethra caused by an organism other than Neisseria gonorrhoeae.

Non-Hodgkins Lymphoma (NHL)
a rare type of cancer of the lymph nodes. NHL is characterised by abnormal growth of B-cells and is the most common type of lymphoma in people with HIV/AIDS.

Non-Nucleoside Reverse Transcriptase Inhibitor
a drug (e.g., nevirapine, delavirdine) that inhibits the action of the HIV-1 reverse transcriptase enzyme, thus blocking HIV replication, yet works in a different way than nucleoside analog drugs, by binding with the RT enzyme.

nonopioid analgesic
a pain reliever, e.g., aspirin, ibuprofen, not derived from opium and does not have opium-like characteristics and effects.

nonoxynol-9
a surfactant chemical that is used as a spermicide and microbicide, e.g. in contraceptive foams, as a lubricant on condoms.

non-specific immunity
immune system function, e.g. phagocytosis, that is not directed towards a specific antigen or pathogen. Contrast with specific immunity.

Non-Steroidal Anti-Inflammatory Drug (NSAID)
a drug, e.g. aspirin, ibuprofen that relieves pain and reduces inflammation and fever, but which is not a steroid or a narcotic.

norplant
a progesterone-releasing contraceptive that is embedded under the skin of the upper arm.

nosocomial
refers to the acquisition of a new disease or condition within a healthcare setting, for example a hospital-acquired infection.

NSF
see **National Science Foundation.**

NSI
non-syncytium-inducing strain of HIV.

■ **nucleic acid**

DNA and RNA, molecules made up of nucleotides that carry genetic information.

■ **nucleic acid base**

one of the components that make up the genetic material. In combination with sugar and phosphate groups, they form nucleotides, the 'building blocks' of DNA and RNA. There are two types of bases, purines (adenine and guanine) and pyrmidines (cytosine, thymine and uracil). Bases are complementary and can bind with their counterpart in a process known as base-pairing.

■ **Nucleic Acid Sequence-Based Amplification (NASBA)**

an load assay for detecting HIV viral load in blood plasma. NASBA amplifies RNA rather than DNA.

■ **nucleoside**

a precursor compound that is a converted to a nucleotide by the addition of a phosphate group.

■ **Nucleoside Analog (NA)**

a compound (e.g., AZT, ddI, ddC, d4T, 3TC) that mimics one of the building blocks of DNA and RNA. These compounds suppress retroviral replication by interfering with the reverse transcriptase enzyme. The defective synthetic nucleosides cause premature termination of the viral DNA chain. Nucleoside analogs are prodrugs that are converted into active agents by phosphorylation.

■ **nucleotide**

one of the building blocks that make up the genetic material (DNA and RNA). Nucleotides consist of a base (adenine, cytosine, guanine, thymine or uracil), a sugar and a phosphate group.

■ **nucleotide analog**

a compound (e.g., cidofovir, PMPA), similar to a nucleoside analog, which is already 'primed' with an extra phosphate group and ready to be added to a DNA chain. The defective synthetic nucleotide interferes with viral replication by causing premature termination of the viral DNA chain.

■ **nutrient**

any item that nourishes or promotes growth and metabolism. Nutrients act as cofactors in many vital physiological processes.

nutrition
the processes involved in ingesting and metabolising food material by living plants and animals.

o.d.
pharmaceutical abbreviation, right eye (oculo dextro)

o.s.
pharmaceutical abbreviation, left eye (oculo sinistro)

o.u.
pharmaceutical abbreviation, each eye (oculo utro)

observational study
a study in which no experimental drug is administered, but the patient's symptoms, laboratory values and response to treatment are observed during the course of normal medical management.

obstetrics
the medical specialty concerned with pregnancy and birth.

Occupational Safety And Health Administration (OSHA)
the U.S. federal agency which develops policies and handles enforcement around safety in the workplace.

octoxynol
a surfactant chemical used as a spermicide and microbicide.

ocular
relating to the eye.

Odds Ratio (OR)
a statistical measure of the likelihood of developing a disease or condition if exposed to a certain factor or pathogen.

odynophagia
painful swallowing.

oedema
swelling caused by an abnormal accumulation of fluid in body tissues.

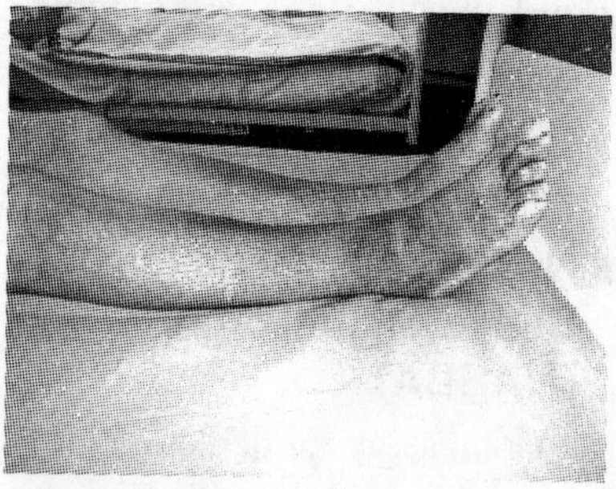

off label use
a drug prescribed for a condition other than the approved conditions.

Office Of Aids Research (OAR)
the U.S. federal agency responsible for coordinating AIDS research done by various federal departments, institutes and agencies.

■ **off-label**
use of an FDA-approved drug for an indication other than that for which the drug was approved.

■ **OHL**
see **oral hairy leukoplakia.**

■ **OI**
abbreviation, opportunistic infection

■ **oligo-**
prefix, few.

■ **oligodendrocyte**
a type of brain cell that produces myelin, a protective covering necessary for proper neural transmission.

■ **oligomenorrhoea**
sparse menstrual bleeding.

■ **oligonucleotide**
a sequence of nucleotides, the building blocks of DNA.

■ **oncogen**
an agent, e.g. virus. toxin that is able to cause neoplastic cell growth or cancer.

■ **oncogene**
a gene e.g. p53 that facilitates the development of cancer by regulating cell growth, either by actively 'turning on' abnormal cell growth or failing to 'turn off' normal cell growth.

■ **oncogenesis**
the development and growth of a tumour.

■ **oncology**
the study and treatment of cancer.

■ **onychomycosis**
a fungal infection that causes the toenails and/or fingernails to thicken, discolour and split. Onychomycosis is often one of the earliest manifestations of HIV disease progression.

■ **oocyst**
the earliest stage of the life cycle of a parasitic protozoan, e.g. cryptosporidium in which it is enclosed in a hard-shelled capsule. Oocysts are dormant (non-growing) but may still be infectious.

■ **oophorectomy**
surgical removal of the ovaries.

■ **oophoritis**
inflammation of the ovaries, a possible manifestation of pelvic inflammatory disease.

■ **open label trial**
a clinical trial of a drug where researchers and patients know which drug is being administered.

■ **open trial**
a clinical trial of a drug where

researchers and patients know which drug is being administered.

open-label

refers to a drug trial which is not randomised and not blinded. Both participants and investigators know what drug is being tested and what dose is being used.

ophthalmic

pertaining to the eye.

ophthalmology

the medical specialty relating to the treatment of diseases and disorders of the eye.

opiate antagonist

an agent e.g. naltrexone that binds to the body's opiate receptors thereby blocking the activity of opioid drugs, e.g. heroin and endorphins.

opiate receptor

molecular structures on the cells that respond to or are influenced by opiate and endorphin molecules. Opiate receptors are found on certain types of cells in the brain, lungs, pancreas, endocrine glands and other organs and tissues.

opioid

a class of drugs, e.g. heroin, codeine, methadone that are derived from the opium poppy plant, contain opium or are produced synthetically and have opium-like effects. Opioid drugs relieve pain, dull the senses and induce sleep.

Opportunistic Infection (OI)

an illness caused by a micro-organism that usually does not cause disease in persons with healthy immune systems, but which may cause serious illness when the immune system is suppressed. Common OI in HIV positive people include Pneumocystis carinii pneumonia (PCP), Mycobacterium avium complex (MAC) and cytomegalovirus (CMV) infection.

oral

relating to the mouth or taken by mouth.

oral candidiasis (thrush)

a fungal infection of the mouth, usually caused by Candida albicans, which typically appears as white or red patches on the oral mucosa, tongue, palate or back of the throat. Types include pseudomembranous candidiasis (thrush), characterised by removable white plaques, acute atrophic candidiasis and chronic atrophic candidiasis (angular cheilitis).

■ **oral hairy leukoplakia**
a condition believed to be caused by the Epstein-Barr virus characterised by white, raised, usually painless lesions on the sides of the tongue and/or elsewhere in the mouth.

■ **organomegaly**
enlargement or swelling of an organ.

■ **oropharynx (adjective oropharyngeal)**
the central portion of the pharynx (throat), between the soft palate and the epiglottis.

■ **orphan drug act**
a law designed to facilitate the development of drugs to treat rare disorders, by providing financial incentives to drug companies.

■ **orthopaedics**
the branch of medicine that deals with preserving and restoring function of the musculo-skeletal system using physical or surgical methods.

■ **os**
the opening of the uterine cervix into the vagina.

■ **osteomyelitis**
an inflammation of the bone and/or bone marrow.

■ **osteoporosis**
atrophy of the bone tissue; loss of calcium from the bones. Osteoporosis is influenced by hormonal levels and may be ameliorated by adequate calcium intake.

■ **otitis media**
inflammation of the middle ear.

■ **otolaryngology (ENT)**
the medical specialty concerned with the ears, nose and throat.

■ **outbreak**
a recurrence of a latent infection (e.g. a herpes simplex virus outbreak). Also refers to the widespread occurrence of a disease within a population.

■ **outpatient**
a patient who is treated outside a hospital or other medical facility.

■ **ovary**
one of the 2 female gonads located within the abdomen on either side of the uterus. The ovaries are the site of egg (ova) storage and maturation.

■ **over-the-counter (otc)**
drugs that are available without a prescription.

■ **oviduct**
see **fallopian tube.**

■ **ovum (plural ova)**
an egg.

■ **oxandrolone**
an anabolic (mass-building) steroid that may lack some of the hormonal side effects of testosterone. The drug is under study as a therapy for HIV wasting syndrome.

■ **oxidation**
a chemical reaction in which another substance combines with oxygen by giving up an electron. Oxidants (pro-oxidants) promote this reaction, while antioxidants inhibit it. Oxidation is the process by which carbohydrates, fats and proteins from food are broken down to provide usable energy for the body.

■ **oxidative stress**
increased levels of free radicals and other oxidation-promoting molecules associated with disease, immune response and aging. When the production of pro-oxidants exceeds the cellular supply of antioxidants, harmful effects may result including cell membrane damage, cell death and damage to genetic material (DNA and RNA) resulting in mutations.

■ **oxygenated blood**
blood that has passed through the lungs and exchanged its carbon dioxide for oxygen. Oxygenated blood is pumped from the left ventricle to the various organs and tissues of the body.

■ **ozone**
a reactive form of oxygen containing 3 atoms. Ozone is capable of killing many pathogens and may be used as a germicide (e.g., in water treatment).

■ **ozonization**
the addition of ozone for disinfectant purposes.

■ **p.**
pharmaceutical abbreviation, after (post).

■ **p.c.**
pharmaceutical abbreviation, after meals (*post cibum*).

■ **p.o.**
pharmaceutical abbreviation, taken by mouth.

■ **p.r.n.**
pharmaceutical abbreviation, as necessary (*pro re nata*).

■ **p24**
a core protein of HIV produced by the gag gene.

■ **p24 antibody**
antibodies produced in response

to the presence of p24 antigen of HIV. The p24 antibody test measures the level of p24 antibodies in the blood. High levels of p24 antibody in the absence of p24 antigen may indicate that the immune system is successfully suppressing the virus.

■ **p24 antigen**
protein fragment (nucleocapsid) of HIV. At one time, p24 antigen was considered a surrogate marker for disease progression. Today, scientists know there are long-term non-progressors with high p24 lab readings. Others have died of AIDS without ever showing any p24 antigen.

■ **p450**
see **cytochrome P450 system.**

■ **paclitaxel**
a drug derived from the yew tree that is used to treat certain types of cancer, e.g. ovarian cancer. Paclitaxel works by inhibiting cell division and is under study for the treatment of Kaposi's sarcoma.

■ **palliative**
offering symptomatic relief and comfort care, e.g. alleviation of pain rather than a cure.

■ **palpitation**
pulsation of the heart, usually with an increase in force or frequency of the heartbeat.

■ **panacea**
a miracle cure-all.

■ **pancreas**
a gland lying behind the stomach that creates insulin and pancreatic juice — a clear, alkaline containing enzymes used during digestion.

■ **pancreatitis**
potentially fatal inflammation of the pancreas. Pancreatitis is a side effect of some anti-HIV drugs. Symptoms include severe stomach pain.

■ **pancytopenia**
low levels of all types of blood cells.

■ **pandemic**
a widespread disease outbreak affecting the population of an extensive area of the world. See also **epidemic.**

■ **papanicolaou smear (pap smear)**
a procedure in which a specimen of cells is taken from the uterine cervix or anus, prepared on a slide and examined under a microscope for abnormal cell growth (dysplasia). An abnormal Pap smear suggests increased risk

of developing cancer.

papillomavirus
see **human papillomavirus.**

papovavirus
a type of virus that can cause neoplasms, e.g. warts, cancer.

papule
a small raised bump on the skin or mucous membrane.

para-
prefix, beside, near.

Paracocc idioidomycosis
a fungal infection endemic to South and Central America. The disease develops in the lungs and may become chronic in immunosuppressed individuals.

paradigm
a theoretical framework that forms the basis for hypotheses and explanations.

parallel track
a system of making experimental drugs available to individuals who are ineligible for or unable to participate in clinical trials. Parallel track drugs have completed Phase I safety testing and show enough evidence of efficacy to merit wider release.

paranasal sinus
an air-filled cavity within the skull; there are 4 sets of paranasal sinuses: frontal, maxillary, sphenoidal and ethmoid.

paraplegia
paralysis of both legs and the lower part of the body. See also **quadriplegia.**

parasite
an organism that grows and feeds in or on another organism without benefiting the host organism. Most parasites are harmless, but some are deadly. The most common ways of getting a parasitic infection are from contaminated water and rimming (oral-anal contact).

parasympathetic nervous system
a branch of the autonomic nervous system that tends to induce secretion, increase the tone and contraction of smooth muscle and cause dilation of blood vessels.

parenchyma
the internal functional tissues of an organ, as opposed to supporting or structural tissues.

parenteral
given by injection, bypassing the enteral (gastrointestinal) tract.

parenteral nutrition
a regimen that delivers nutrients intravenously, bypassing the gas-

trointestinal tract. Partial Parenteral Nutrition (PPN) delivers some nutrients orally and some intravenously, total parenteral nutrition (TPN) delivers all nutrient intravenously, typically into a large central vein via a chest catheter.

■ **paresthesia**
abnormal physical sensations such as prickling or tingling.

■ **parkinson's disease (parkinsonism)**
a chronic progressive nerve disease characterised by muscle tremors, weakness, rigid movements, halting gait, drooping posture and expressionless facial appearance.

■ **paromomycin (humatin)**
an antibiotic used to treat intestinal infections, such as amebiasis and giardiasis and under study as a treatment for cryptosporidiosis.

■ **paronychia**
inflammation and separation of the skin from the base of the nails.

■ **parotitis**
inflammation of the parotid gland, the largest of the salivary glands.

■ **Partial Parenteral Nutrition (PPN)**
see **arenteral nutrition.**

■ **parvovirus**
a family of viruses, several species of which infect humans, including the adeno-associated viruses which are used as vectors in biotechnology. Parvoviruses tend to infect rapidly growing tissues. Symptoms include fever, malaise and possibly skin rash.

■ **Passive Hyperimmune Therapy (PHT)**
an experimental treatment for HIV infection that involves monthly infusions of p24 antibody-rich plasma (hyperimmune plasma) from asymptomatic healthy HIV positive donors to patients with advanced HIV disease.

■ **passive immunity**
immunity acquired by transfer of antibodies, either naturally (e.g., from mother to foetus) or by injection. Contrast with active immunity.

■ **passive immunisation (passive immunotherapy)**
the introduction of exogenous antibodies i.e. gamma globulins to treat disease, for example from an individual with active immunity or of genetically engineering antibodies. Contrast with active immunisation.

pasteurisation
partial sterilisation of a substance, especially a liquid, using heat to destroy harmful organisms without inducing major chemical alteration of the substance.

pastille
a lozenge, a medicated disc or tablet dissolved in the mouth.

pathogen (adjective pathogenic)
any disease-causing agent, especially a micro-organism.

pathogenesis
the development of a particular disease, including the specific events involved, bodily tissues or systems affected, mechanisms of damage and timing of the course of disease.

pathogenicity
the property of being able to cause disease.

pathology (adjective pathologic)
the study of disease, focusing on causes, development and progress of disease and how the body is affected.

PBMC
see **Peripheral Blood Mononuclear Cell.**

pcg
pharmaceutical abbreviation, picogram.

pcp
abbreviation, pneumocystis carinii pneumonia, a fungal inflammation of the lungs. PCP was once the leading cause of death of people with HIV Disease. Today it is still dangerous but is often treatable and preventable.

PCR
see **Polymerase Chain Reaction.**

peak level
the highest concentration of a drug achieved in the body.

pediatrics
the medical specialty concerned with the development, care and treatment of children from birth through adolescence.

pediculosis
lice infestation.

pelvic exam
examination of the organs of the female reproductive system. A speculum is used to open the vagina and aid in visualising the uterine cervix; a sample of cells may be taken for a Pap smear or laboratory culture. The uterus and ovaries are palpated i.e.felt with the fingers to detect swellings or other abnormalities.

Pelvic Inflammatory Disease (PID)
infection of the upper female reproductive tract including the uterus, fallopian tubes and ovaries. PID is often the result of untreated chlamydiasis or gonorrhea. Symptoms include pain, fever and vaginal discharge. Without treatment, PID can become chronic and severe and may lead to scarring, infertility, ectopic pregnancy, septicemia and death.

penicillin
an antibiotic drug used to treat various bacterial infections. Penicillin G is a strong form of penicillin used to treat neurosyphilis.

pentamidine
a drug used to prevent and treat Pneumocystis carinii pneumonia. Intravenous pentamidine is used to treat severe cases of PCP, especially in patients who cannot tolerate TMP-SMX. Aerosolised pentamidine is used as a prophylaxis against PCP. Side effects may include pancreatitis.

pentoxifylline
a drug used to treat circulatory problems. PTX increases the production of interferons and reduces levels of tumour necrosis factor (TNF) in the body.

peptic ulcer
a lesion in the stomach wall caused by infection with the bacterium Heliobacter pylori.

peptide
a short chain of amino acids linked by peptide bonds; longer chains are generally called proteins.

peptide T
a peptide composed of a sequence of 8 amino acids. Peptide T is under study as therapy for HIV-related dementia and peripheral neuropathy.

percutaneous
through the skin.

perianal
refers to the area surrounding the anus.

pericarditis
inflammation of the pericardium, the membrane that surrounds the heart.

perinatal
refers to the period around the time of birth.

Perinatal HIV Transmission (PHT)
the transmission of HIV from a mother to a foetus or infant. An estimated 10-40% of mothers transmit HIV to their offspring. AZT has been shown to significantly reduce the risk of PHT.

periodontal disease (periodontitis)
an inflammatory disease of the tissues that surround and support the teeth. Periodontal disease may begin as gingivitis and progress to more serious gum disease accompanied by erosion of the gums and bone supporting the teeth.

peripheral
pertaining to or located at the periphery or away from the centre.

Peripheral Blood Mononuclear Cell (PBMC)
a single-nucleus white blood cell, e.g. monocyte, that circulates in the blood. See also **mononuclear cell.**

Peripheral Nervous System (PNS)
the portion of the nervous system outside of the brain and spinal cord, PNS includes cranial nerves, spinal nerves and the sympathetic nervous system, i.e. nerves that run from the spinal cord to the rest of the body.

peripheral neuropathy
any disease, inflammation or abnormality of the peripheral nervous system. This is considered as an AIDS-defining condition.

peritoneum
the thick membrane that lines the abdominal cavity and covers the visceral organs. The peritoneal cavity is the space between the outer and inner layers of the peritoneal membrane.

peritonitis
inflammation of the peritoneum.

Persistent Generalised Lymphadenopathy (PGL)
a condition in which the lymph nodes are chronically swollen in more than one area of the body for a prolonged time, sometimes accompanied by a swollen spleen.

ph
a logarithmic scale used to describe the acidity or alkalinity of a solution. A measure of the hydrogen concentration of a solution. Water has a neutral pH of 7. A pH below 7 is acidic, a pH above 7 is alkaline (or basic).

phagocyte
a scavenger white blood cell (e.g., neutrophil, basophil, eosinophil, monocyte, macrophage) that engulfs and destroys dead cells, bacteria and other debris. Once the foreign matter is ingested, phagocytes produce toxic chemicals

(e.g., hydrogen peroxide) to kill the invader.

■ **phagocytosis**
the process of engulfing and destroying matter (e.g., micro-organisms, dead cells) carried out by phagocytes.

■ **pharmaceutical**
refers to the development and manufacture of drugs.

■ **pharmaco-**
prefix, related to drugs or medicine.

■ **pharmacodynamics**
the study of drug activity.

■ **pharmacokinetic trials**
a clinical trial of an experimental drug that concentrates on the body's ability to absorb the drug. Blood tests are commonly given every few minutes or hours during a pharmacokinetic trial.

■ **pharmacokinetics**
the study of drug absorption and metabolism.

■ **pharmacology**
the science of drugs, their sources and how they work. It also studies the specialty of preparing and dispensing drugs.

■ **pharmacotherapy**
the use of drugs to treat disease.

■ **pharyngitis**
pain and inflammation of the pharynx (throat).

■ **pharynx (adjective pharyngeal)**
the throat. The upper part of the gastrointestinal tract between the oral cavity and the oesophagus.

■ **Phase I Clinical Trial**
the first stage of human testing of a new drug, the first clinical trial of an experimental drug, designed to evaluate toxicity (adverse reactions) at various dosing levels. Most phase one clinical trials have only a small number of participants(less than 100) of healthy volunteers. Phase I clinical trials are part of the U.S. FDA approval process.

■ **Phase II Clinical Trial**
the second clinical trial of an experimental drug, designed to evaluate the drug's effectiveness in humans. Drugs that fail phase one never make it to phase two. This second clinical trial usually involves 300 or fewer volunteers. Phase II trials may be divided into Phase IIa (pilot trials in patients with the disease to be treated) and phase IIb (well-controlled efficacy trials).

Phase III Study
the third and final clinical trial of an experimental drug. This third stage in a new drug's approval process expands the test to several thousand volunteers. The purpose is to evaluate the drug in a larger population to make sure the results of the first two phases hold true in a larger base. Problems involving drug interactions commonly surface during this third stage. Phase III trials may compare the drug being tested to other therapies or to placebo. Phase IIIa trials are conducted prior to the filing of a new drug application (NDA); Phase IIIb trials are conducted after an NDA is submitted.

Phase IV Trial
postmarketing studies done after regulatory approval has been granted and the drug has been offered for sale. These trials provide additional information about safety and efficacy in large numbers of patients under 'real world' conditions of use.

phosphorylation
the addition of a phosphate group to a compound by an enzyme, e.g. thymidine kinase, tyrosine kinase. Phosphorylation is an essential step in many cellular processes.

Photodynamic Therapy (PDT)
a form of cancer treatment in which a patient is exposed to light, e.g. ultraviolet light, light from a laser after ingesting a light-sensitive chemical, e.g. hematoporphyrin, which accumulates in tumour tissue.

photophobia
excessive sensitivity to light.

photosensitivity
an increased sensitivity to light, which may lead to easy sun burning and other adverse effects. Photosensitivity is a side effect of some drugs, e.g. dapsone, hypericin.

phototherapy
treatment using light, typically ultraviolet light.

PHT
see **Passive Hyperimmune Therapy, Perinatal HIV Transmission.**

Physicians' Desk Reference (PDR)
a book of prescription drugs and their indications for use.

pi
see **Principle Investigator, Protease Inhibitor.**

pico-
prefix, one-trillionth.

■ **PID**

see **Pelvic Inflammatory Disease.**

■ **pigment**

organic colouring matter; the chemicals in the skin, eyes, etc. that give a particular colour.

■ **pituitary gland**

a small gland in the brain that produces several hormones that regulate bodily functions via the action of other endocrine glands.

■ **placebo**

an inactive substance given to a control group in a clinical trial. This placebo is sometimes called a sugar pill because some of these control groups are given common substances, such as sugar, disguised as medication.

■ **placebo effect**

a change, e.g. a reduction in symptoms, that is attributable to the treatment process itself as opposed to the therapeutic value of the agents or therapies used, most likely due to the expectations of the patient.

■ **Placebo-Controlled Clinical Trial**

a clinical trial in which one group of volunteers is given the experimental drug and the other group is given a placebo. The results of the two groups are compared to see if the experimental drug was effective compared to the placebo. In many HIV-related clinical trials, some approved treatment is used instead of a placebo.

■ **placenta**

the vascular organ that connects the foetus and the mother's uterus, through which metabolic exchange between the foetus and mother occurs. Some pathogenic organisms and maternal antibodies may be transferred across the placenta.

■ **plasma**

the fluid, non-cellular portion of circulating blood that carries blood cells and nutrients throughout the body, removes metabolic wastes and is a medium for chemical communications between different parts of the body.

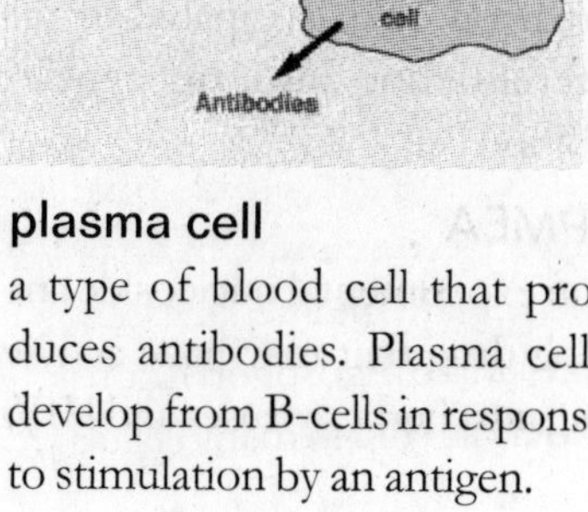

■ **plasma cell**

a type of blood cell that produces antibodies. Plasma cells develop from B-cells in response to stimulation by an antigen.

plasmapheresis
the selective removal of components from the blood plasma, after which the plasma is returned to the person from which it was taken.

platelet
a small blood cell (protoplasmic disk) involved in coagulation and wound healing. HIV can lower a person's platelet count, causing severe bleeding. The normal platelet count is 200,000 to 300,000.

pleura
the linings of the lung.

pleurisy
swelling of the linings of the lung characterised by pain and shortness of breath.

pleuritis
inflammation of the pleura or linings of the lung.

pluripotent stem cell
a haematopoietic cell in the bone marrow that is capable of differentiating into any type of blood cell.

PMEA
an experimental nucleoside analog drug that may have activity against herpes viruses and HIV.

PML
abbreviation, Progressive Multifocal Leukoencephalopathy. a viral infection of the brain. Symptoms include memory loss, loss of strength, coma and death.

PMPA
an experimental nucleotide analog, related to PMEA. PMPA can enter infected as well as uninfected cells.

PMS
see **Premenstrual Syndrome.**

pneumococcus
the organism that causes pneumococcal pneumonia.

Pneumocystis Carinii Pneumonia (PCP)
1. a fungal inflammation of the lungs, commonly abbreviated PCP. PCP was once the leading cause of death of people with HIV Disease. Today it is still dangerous but is often treatable and preventable. PCP is considered an AIDS-defining condition.
2. a life-threatening type of pneumonia believed to be caused by a protozoan. PCP is a common infection that can cause severe illness in immunocompromised people (especially those with CD4 counts less than 200 cells/mm3). It remains a leading cause

of death in people with AIDS. Symptoms include dry cough, fever, chest tightness and shortness of breath. Pneumocystis carinii can also infect other parts of the body. First-line treatment and primary prophylaxis is TMP-SMX (Bactrim, Septra). Other treatments and prophylaxes include dapsone, pentamidine and atovaquone.

■ pneumonia
a group of diseases that show up as an inflammation of the lungs. Recurrent pneumonia (pneumonia recurring within 1 year) is considered as an AIDS-defining condition.

■ pneumonitis
an inflammation of the lungs. The disease pneumonia is on type of pneumonitis.

■ pneumovax vaccine
a vaccine developed to prevent pneumonia caused by common pneumococcal strains.

■ po
given by mouth (*Latin per os*).

■ pol
the HIV gene that encodes the replicative enzymes (protease, integrase, reverse transcriptase). Also the protein produced by that gene.

■ poly-
prefix, many.

■ polycythemia
abnormally high level of red blood cells in the circulating blood.

■ polymerase
an enzyme that cleaves polymers, chemical compounds formed by the linkage of molecular pieces.

■ Polymerase Chain Reaction Assay (PCR)
a sensitive lab test to determine a patient's viral load. It works by repeatedly copying genetic material using heat cycling and enzymes. A viral load test is used to see how well a drug regimen is working. The lower the viral load the better.

■ polymicrobial
including or caused by more than one micro-organism.

■ Polymorphonuclear Leukocyte (PMNL)
a type of white blood cell, e.g. neutrophil containing more than one nucleus. PMNL are phagocytes (scavenger cells) important in immune defence, particularly against cell-free organisms such as fungi.

polyneuropathy
a type of peripheral neuropathy that involves damage to multiple nerves of the peripheral nervous system. Demyelinating polyneuropathy which involves the destruction of the myelin sheath surrounding the neurons and sensory axonal polyneuropathy are common in people with HIV disease. Symptoms may include weakness and painful tingling or burning sensations. See also peripheral neuropathy.

polyp
any mass of tissue that bulges or projects outward or upward from the normal surface level. A polyp may be a precursor to cancer.

polyprotein
a long thread of proteins produced during viral replication. The polyprotein is broken down by the protease enzyme into smaller components, which are then assembled into new virus particles.

polyradiculopathy
a type of peripheral neuropathy characterised by the inflammation of the nerve roots.

polysaccharide
a carbohydrate compound made up of 2 or more sugar molecules. A component of the capsules of fungi.

Positron Emission Tomography (PET) Scan
a method of imaging the brain by recording activity, as measured by cerebral blood flow, in different parts.

post hoc
after the fact.

post mortem
after death, a post mortem examination is an autopsy.

Post-Herpetic Neuralgia (PHN)
the often severe pain along a nerve pathway that sometimes follows the healing of herpes zoster (shingles) lesions.

post-marketing study
see Phase IV trial.

postnatal
the period following birth.

postpartum
the period following childbirth.

potentiation
an increase in activity or effectiveness; an interaction between drugs that results in a synergistic effect.

poxvirus
one of a large family of viruses,

e.g. smallpox that typically cause skin eruptions.

■ **PPD test (mantoux test)**
a test that uses an injection of a purified protein derivative of tuberculin to test for prior exposure to Mycobacterium tuberculosis. A positive reaction is indicated by induration i.e. redness and swelling at the injection site, but it does not mean you have the disease.

■ **preclinical testing**
testing of an experimental drug in the laboratory or in animals prior to testing in humans.

■ **prednisone**
a corticosteroid drug with immunosuppressive effects that is used to decrease inflammation. Side effect may include mood changes, nausea and high blood pressure.

■ **pre-existing condition**
a medical problem that existed before or a specific date.

■ **premalignant**
refers to cells that display abnormal growth and development and may be an early stage in the development of cancer.

■ **Premenstrual Syndrome (PMS)**
a set of symptoms occurring before or during the menstrual period, characterised by cramps, fatigue, bloating and mood changes.

■ **prenatal**
the period preceding birth, during which the foetus develops in the uterus.

■ **presumptive diagnosis/ treatment**
treatment based on an assumed diagnosis, prior to receiving confirmatory laboratory test results.

■ **prevalence (prevalence rate)**
the number of individuals with a condition in a specific population. The prevalence rate is determined by dividing the number of people with the condition by the total population.

■ **preventive vaccine (prophylactic vaccine)**
a vaccine that is intended to prevent a disease from occurring by priming the immune system to respond to a pathogenic organism. Contrast with therapeutic vaccine.

■ **primary central nervous system lymphoma**
a malignant proliferation of B-cells in the central nervous system associated with the Epstein-

Barr virus. Symptoms include partial paralysis, aphasia, lethargy, confusion, memory loss and seizures.

■ primary HIV infection
the initial stage of infection with HIV, prior to the development of antibodies. Primary HIV infection may be accompanied by acute retroviral syndrome, characterised by flu-like symptoms including fever, malaise, enlarged lymph glands, sore throat, skin rash and muscle and/or joint aches.

■ primary infection
the initial introduction of an infectious organism into the body.

■ primary prophylaxis
a treatment intended to prevent the first occurrence of an infection or disease. Contrast with secondary prophylaxis.

■ principal neutralising determinant
the part of an antigen that most reliably induces a protective immune response. The principal neutralising determinant of HIV is the V3 loop of the envelope glycoprotein gp120.

■ principle investigator
the chief researcher in a clinical trial.

■ prn
administered as needed (*Latin pro re nata*).

■ probenicid
a drug that promotes metabolism by the liver and kidneys and which may be given with other drugs to lessen liver and/or kidney toxicity.

■ proctitis
inflammation of the mucous membranes of the rectum.

■ proctoscopy
examination of the rectum and lower end of the colon with a lighted instrument.

■ prodrome
a set of symptoms or signs, e.g. itching, tingling, pain that indicate the onset of a disease, e.g. a herpes simplex outbreak.

■ prodrug
an inactive form of a drug that exerts its effects after metabolic changes within the body convert it to a usable or active form.

■ progesterone
a female steroid hormone with anti-estrogen effects. Progesterone prepares the uterus for the development of the fertilised ovum and maintains the uterus throughout pregnancy. Synthetic

progesterone is used as a contraceptive.

■ **progestin**
a hormone produced by the corpus luteum, placenta or adrenal cortex that has progesterone-like effects. Synthetic progestin is used as a contraceptive.

■ **prognosis (adjective prognostic)**
a forecast of the probable course and/or outcome of a disease.

■ **programmed cell death**
see **apoptosis**.

■ **progressive disease**
a disease that continually increases in severity.

■ **Progressive Multifocal Leukoencephalopathy (PML)**
a rapidly progressing, often fatal brain disease believed to be caused by the Jacob-Creutzfeldt (JC) papovavirus. PML infects oligodendrocytes (support cells in the brain) and leads to dysfunctional nerve signal transmission. Symptoms include headaches, changes in mental status, speech and vision difficulties, limb weakness, seizures, partial paralysis and loss of coordination.

■ **proinflammatory cytokine**
a chemical messenger, e.g. IL-1, IL-6, tumour necrosis factor produced by the body that promotes an inflammatory immune response.

■ **prokinetic antiemetic**
a drug that relieves nausea by promoting gastrointestinal motility or speeds up the digestive and excretory processes.

■ **prolactin**
a pituitary hormone that stimulates the secretion of breast milk.

■ **proleukin**
see **interleukin 2.**

■ **proliferation**
rapid or uncontrolled reproduction or replication.

■ **prophylaxis**
1. a defence or protection. Several drugs are available for patients with suppressed immune systems to prevent certain opportunistic infections. For example, Bactrim is a prophylaxis against PCP. Using a condom is a phophylaxis against most sexually transmitted diseases.
2. a treatment that helps to prevent a disease or condition before it occurs (primary prophylaxis) or recurs (secondary prophylaxis).

■ **prospective study**

a study that looks forward in time. Patients are selected and their progression is followed. A prospective cohort study follows a specific group of people over a period of time. Contrast with retrospective study.

■ **prostaglandin**

a locally-acting chemical messenger that is produced by many types of cells. Prostaglandins have a wide variety of effects including vasodilation and smooth muscle regulation. Prostaglandins have a role in allergic reactions, uterine contraction, inflammation and pain signalling.

■ **prostate gland**

a large gland in males located at the base of the urethra that manufactures the liquid portion of semen.

■ **protease**

an enzyme that breaks down proteins and is used in cell replication. There are many kinds of protease, most of which are beneficial. One enzyme is specific to the HIV replication process.

■ **protease**

an enzyme that cleaves proteins. HIV protease cleaves the large precursor proteins produced from viral RNA into the component parts that are then assembled into new viral particles. Protease is essential for the production of infectious new virions.

■ **protease inhibitor**

a class of anti-HIV drug that prevents creation of an HIV-specific protease.

■ **proteinase**

see **protease**.

■ **proteinuria**

the abnormal presence of protein in the urine.

■ **Prothrombin Time (PT)**

a test that measures blood coagulation ability. Prothrombin is a protein produced by the liver that facilitates blood clotting.

■ **provirus**

a viral state in which viral DNA has been inserted into the chromosome of the host cell.

■ **pruritus (adjective pruritic)**

a condition characterised by itching.

■ **pseudomembranous candidiasis**

see **oral candidiasis.**

■ **pseudomeningitis**

see **meningismus.**

■ **pseudomonas**

a group of aerobic rod-shaped bacteria, some of which, e.g. P. aeruginosa, P. flourescens, can cause opportunistic infections in human.

■ **psoriasis**

a common chronic skin condition characterised by reddish scaly patches, primarily on the scalp, elbows, knees and trunk. Outbreaks are more common and may be more severe in HIV-infected individuals. Psoriatic arthritis is a form of arthritis accompanied by psoriasis.

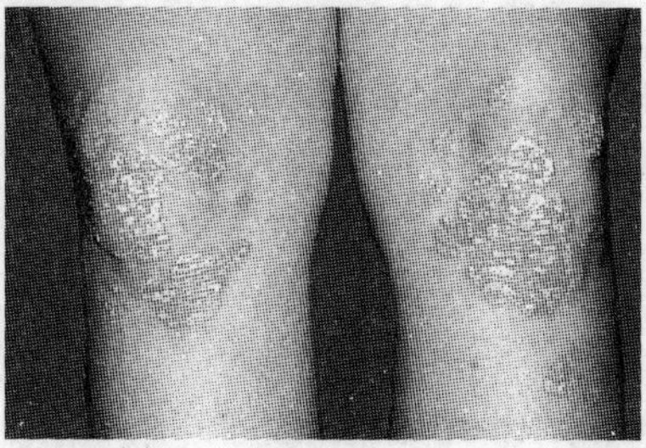

■ **psychomotor**

relating to mental functioning and control of muscular movement.

■ **Psychoneuroimmunology (PNI)**

the study of how psychological processes, mental state and neurological and hormonal factors affect the functioning of the immune system.

■ **psychopharmacology**

the use of drugs that affect the psyche or personality.

■ **psychosis**

a major mental disorder (e.g., schizophrenia, bipolar disorder) that affects the ability to function normally on a daily basis.

■ **psychosocial**

refers to factors that affect the psychological or social realm. Psychosocial factors, e.g. socioeconomic status, education, family situation, may make an important contribution to disease risk and progression and are an essential aspect of a person's wellbeing.

■ **psychotropic**

an agent, e.g. thorazine that affects psychic or mental functioning or behaviour.

■ **Public Health Service (PHS)**

the U.S. federal agency, part of the Department of Health and Human Services, that oversees the health of the public, monitors epidemics, etc. The National Institutes of Health (NIH) and the Centres for Disease Control and Prevention (CDC) are part of the PHS.

■ **puerperal sepsis (puerperal fever)**
an infection, e.g. with Streptococcus bacteria acquired during childbirth. Puerperal fever is an outcome of puerperal sepsis characterised by fever, rapid heartbeat and inflammation of the uterus. The condition may be fatal.

■ **pulmonary**
relating to the lungs.

■ **pulse oximetry**
a method of measuring the amount of oxygen in the blood by means of a clip-like instrument that attaches to the finger.

■ **punch biopsy**
the removal of a small piece of tissue from the skin or mucous membrane for diagnostic analysis.

■ **purine**
one of the 2 types of nucleotide bases that make up DNA and RNA. The purine bases are adenine and guanine. See also **pyrimidine.**

■ **purpura**
a purplish discoloration due to bleeding underneath the skin.

■ **purulent**
characterised by the accumulation of pus.

■ **pus**
a thick, greenish-yellow fluid composed of dead white blood cells, killed micro-organisms and other cellular debris.

■ **pustule**
a small skin elevation or blister containing pus.

■ **PWA**
abbreviation, Person with AIDS.

■ **PWHIV**
person or people with HIV infection.

■ **px**
medical abbreviation for preventive therapy or prophylaxis.

■ **pyridoxine (vitamin b6)**
a form of vitamin B that helps prevent peripheral neuropathy side effects when used with certain drugs, e.g. isoniazid.

■ **pyrimethamine**
a drug used to treat protozoan infections such as toxoplasmosis. Side effects include bone marrow suppression and allergic skin reactions.

■ **pyrimidine**
one of the 2 types of nucleotide base that make up DNA and RNA. The pyrimidine bases are cytosine, thymine and uracil. See also purine.

■ q
medical abbreviation for every, often used to specify drug dosing schedules (e.g., q6h indicates every 6 hours; qiw indicates 4 times per week).

■ q. __ h.
every __ hours (*quaque 4 horae*) 'every four hours'

■ q.d.
every day (*quaque die*).

■ q.i.d
four times a day (*quarter in die*).

■ q.i.w.
four times a week.

■ q.m.
every month.

■ q.o.d.
every other day.

■ q.o.w.
every other week.

■ q.s. ad
a sufficient quantity to make (*quantum sufficiat ad*).

■ qc-pcr
see **quantitative competitive polymerase chain reaction.**

■ qi (chi, xi)
the vital energy believed to be responsible for health and disease in Traditional Chinese Medicine.

■ quadriplegia
paralysis from the neck down, including the trunk and both legs and arms. See also **paraplegia.**

■ qualitative
relating to or expressed in terms of, quality. Qualitative research is based on individual, often subjective, analysis.

■ Quantiplex HIV RNA Assay
see **branched-chain DNA assay.**

■ quantitative
relating to or expressed in terms of, quantity. Quantitative research is based on numerical data.

■ quiescent
refers to a state of resting, inactivity or latency.

■ quinolinic acid
a naturally occurring toxin in the central nervous system, believed to play a role in AIDS dementia complex.

■ r
abbreviation for recombinant.

■ radical
a highly reactive molecule that may pass intact from one compound to another but does not normally exist in a free state. See also **free radical.**

radioimmunoassay
a procedure for detecting antigens or antibodies using radioactive-labelled complement proteins.

radiology
a branch of medicine concerned with the use of X-rays to diagnose and/or treat disease.

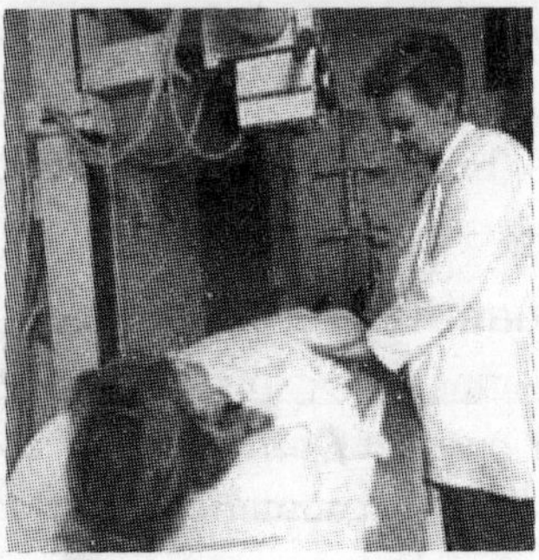

radiotherapy (radiation therapy)
the use of radiation, most often X-rays, to treat cancer or other diseases.

rantes
a chemokine protein that affects HIV activity. RANTES is believed to act in conjunction with 2 other chemokines, MIP-1-alpha and MIP-1-beta.

RAU
Recurrent Aphthous Ulcers. See **aphthous ulcer.**

RBC
Red Blood Cell.

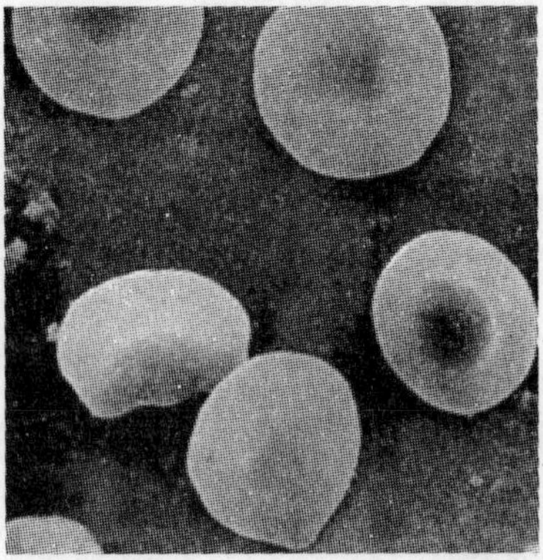

Rd
Registered Dietitian.

RDA
see **recommended daily allowance.**

reactivation
the return of a previously latent (inactive) infection to an active, pathogenic state.

receptor
a specific protein-binding site on a cell's surface or interior. When chemical messengers bind to receptors, various cellular functions are activated or inhibited. Many drugs exert their effects by binding to receptors and altering normal cellular communication. Viruses enter cells by fusing with receptors on the cell surface, often in conjunction with MHC molecules and/or co-receptors.

■ **rechallenge**
to administer the same substance, e.g. pathogenic organism, drug a second or subsequent time. Rechallenge may be done after vaccination to determine whether a vaccine was effective.

■ **recombinant**
produced by genetic engineering. Recombinant products are designated by a lower-case r (e.g. rHGH).

■ **recombinant dna**
genetically engineered DNA (e.g., new DNA produced by joining pieces of DNA from different sources).

■ **Recommended Daily Allowance (RDA)**
the amount of a nutrient that is recommended each day to avoid deficiency diseases.

■ **reconstitution**
rebuilding and restoring to functionality, e.g. reconstitution of a damaged immune system.

■ **recrudescence**
a new outbreak or active replication of a pathogenic organism after a period of inactivity.

■ **rectum (adjective rectal)**
the lower part of the large intestine where faeces are stored.

■ **recurrent**
returning or occurring repeatedly.

■ **refractory**
resistant to treatment.

■ **regimen**
see **dosage regimen**.

■ **rehydration**
replacement of lost fluids.

■ **Reiter's Syndrome (reactive arthritis)**
an autoimmune disorder characterised by the simultaneous occurrence of arthritis, urethritis (inflammation of the urethra) and conjunctivitis (inflammation of the outer membrane of the eye). The syndrome may occur following other diseases such as chlamydiasis or salmonellosis.

■ **relapse**
recurrence of disease symptoms following a period of improvement.

■ **Relative Risk (RR)**
a measure of comparative risk of developing a disease or condition. Statistically, RR is the chance that a person receiving an exposure will develop a condition compared to the chance that a non-exposed person will develop the same condition.

remission
an abatement in the severity of disease symptoms. A period of time during which symptoms are reduced or eliminated.

renal
relating to the kidneys.

renal failure
kidney failure.

repletion
replenishment.

replication
duplication or reproduction.

replicative enzyme
an enzyme that is necessary to the reproductive process.

rescue medication
a strong, short-acting analgesic given to control acute episodes of breakthrough pain in a patient on a continuous pain management regimen.

reservoir
a site where an infectious agent collects and multiplies, e.g. macrophages and lymph nodes are believed to be reservoirs for HIV.

resistance
the ability of a micro-organism to mutate or change its structure in such a way that it loses its sensitivity to a drug. A resistant organism can function and replicate despite the drug's presence.

respiratory
relating to the process of breathing.

reticuloendothelial system
a system that helps the body fight infection and eliminate cellular debris by the action of phagocytic cells, e.g. macrophages, Kupffer cells in the liver and reticular cells of the spleen, bone marrow and lymph nodes.

retina
a light-sensitive membrane lining the inner eyeball. Images are formed on the retina before being transmitted to the brain on the optic nerve.

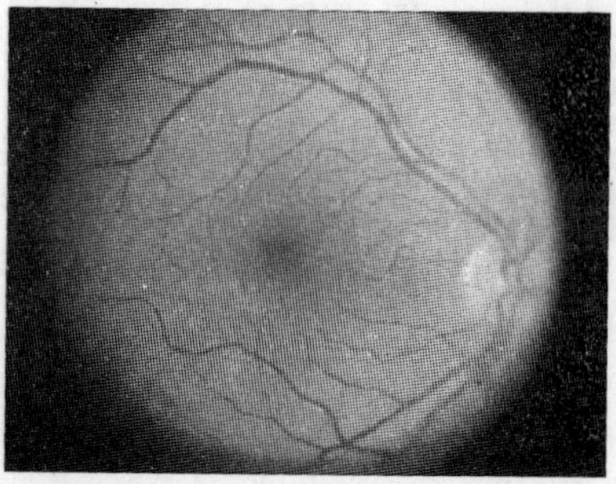

retinal detachment
a condition in which a layer of the retina separates from the underlying epithelium, allowing vitreous fluid to seep behind it. The condition may lead to loss of vision.

retinitis
inflammation of the retina which can lead to blindness.

retinoic acid (retin-a, tretinoin)
a form of vitamin A that stimulates rapid cell turnover and is used to treat severe acne.

retinopathy
any non-inflammatory disease of the retina. Retinopathy is common in people with diabetes.

retrovir
brand name of AZT.

retrovirus
a retrovirus, such as HIV, replicate using an enzyme (reverse transcriptase) to copy RNA into DNA. Most cells have DNA in their natural state and transcribe to RNA during replication. A retrovirus does things backwards — RNA, not DNA, is its natural genetic state. Several anti-HIV drugs — such as AZT, ddI, ddC — are chemicals that act against the reverse transcriptase enzyme.

rev
a gene of HIV; also the protein produced by the gene, which regulates the construction of the structural components of HIV and is necessary for the production of new virus particles.

Reverse Transcriptase (RT)
a viral enzyme that allows a retrovirus to translate its genetic material (in the form of RNA) into DNA, which is then integrated into the chromosomes of the host cell.

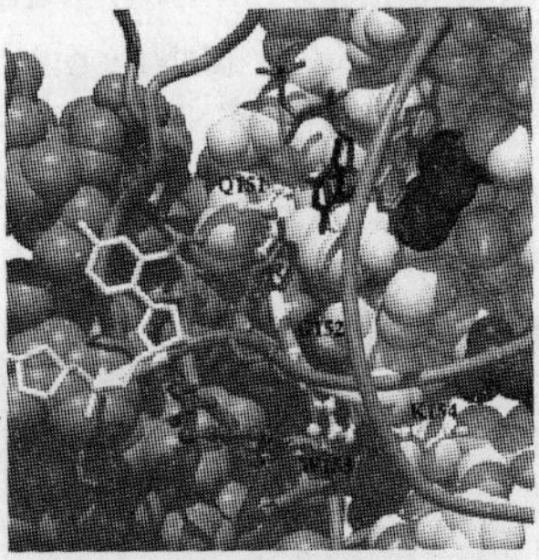

Reverse Transcriptase Inhibitor (RTI)
a drug that blocks retroviral replication by interfering with the reverse transcriptase enzyme. RTI drugs are not effective after a cell has already been infected. RTI drugs include nucleoside analogs, e.g. AZT, ddI, 3TC, d4T and non-nucleoside reverse transcriptase inhibitors, e.g. nevirapine, delavirdine.

rheumatology (adjective rheumatic)
the study of various conditions, e.g. arthritis, polymyositis involving pain or other disorders of the joints.

rhinitis
inflammation of the nasal membranes characterised by sneezing, runny nose and watering eyes, a common manifestation of an allergic reaction.

rhinovirus
one of a large family of viruses that commonly cause respiratory illnesses, characterised by nasal congestion and sore throat, but little or no fever.

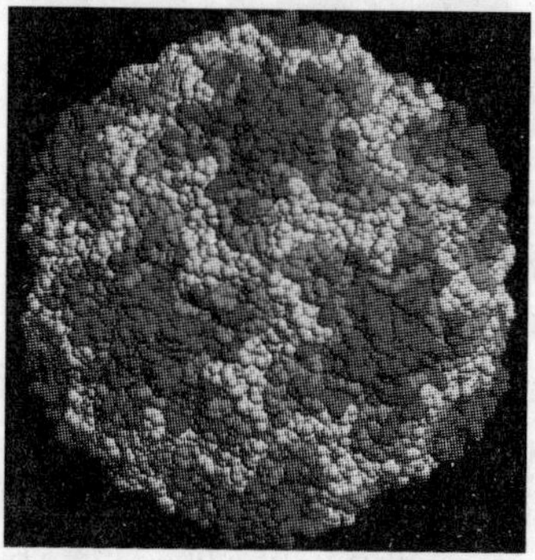

riboflavin (vitamin b2)
see **vitamin B.**

Ribonucleic Acid (RNA)
a single-stranded nucleic acid that encodes genetic information. RNA is made up of sequence of 4 chemical building blocks (nucleotides) — adenine, cytosine, guanine and uracil. RNA is involved in the transcription of genetic information; the information encoded in DNA is translated into messenger RNA (mRNA), which controls the synthesis of new proteins. RNA takes the place of DNA in retroviruses such as HIV. The presence of HIV RNA in the plasma indicates that the virus is actively replicating.

ribonucleotide reductase
a viral enzyme which cuts ribonucleotides in order to create deoxyibonucleotides, the building blocks of DNA. Ribonucleotide reductase is essential for DNA replication.

ribozyme
RNA with enzymatic activity that can break down (cleave) and piece together (splice) genetic material (DNA or RNA), thus modifying the genetic instructions it carries. Ribozymes (e.g., hairpin ribozyme) are used as 'molecular scissors' in genetic engineering.

rifampin
a drug used in combination treatment for tuberculosis and under study for treatment of MAC. Side effects may include orange-coloured body fluids, rash, nausea, fever and liver toxicity.

rimming (analingus)
oral-anal sex. Sexual contact between one person's tongue and/

or mouth and another person's anus.

- **ritonavir (norvir, formerly abt-538)**
  a protease inhibitor drug approved for the treatment of HIV disease. Current practice favours the use of ritonavir in combination therapy (e.g., with nucleoside analog drugs) to avoid the development of drug-resistant virus.
- **roentgenogram**
  a picture produced using X-rays.

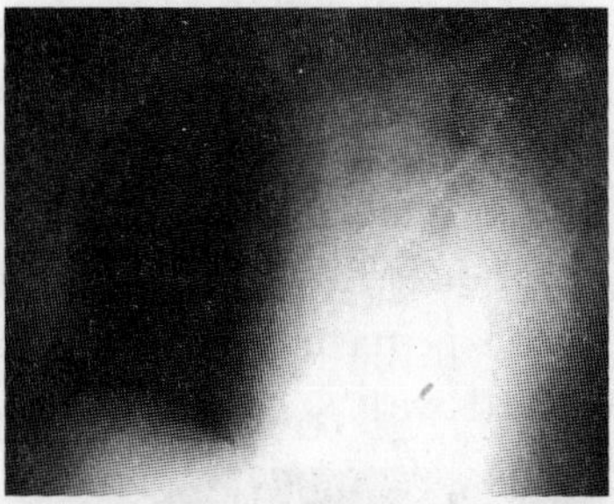

- **roseola**
  see exanthem.
- **RPR test**
  Rapid Plasma Reagin, a blood test for syphilis infection.
- **RT**
  see **reverse transcriptase.**
- **RT-PCR**
  see **Reverse Transcriptase Polymerase Chain Reaction Test.**
- **ru-486**
  a progesterone antagonist drug that has abortifacient (abortion inducing) activity and may inhibit HIV replication.
- **rupture**
  a break or tear of an organ or soft tissues.
- **Rupture of Membranes (ROM)**
  the breaking open of the amniotic sac surrounding the foetus prior to the start of labour and delivery.
- **rx**
  medical abbreviation for prescription.
- **s.o.s.**
  if needed (*si opus sit*).
- **safer sex**
  sexual activities that reduce or eliminate the exchange of body fluids that can transmit HIV (e.g., semen, vaginal or cervical fluid), often by means of barriers (e.g., latex condoms, gloves, dental dams).
- **salmonella septicaemia**
  recurrent salmonella septicemia is considered as an AIDS-defining condition.
- **salmonellosis**
  infection caused by Salmonella,

bacteria commonly found in raw meat, poultry, eggs and raw or unpasteurised milk products. The 3 forms of salmonellosis in humans are typhoid fever, septicaemia (blood poisoning) and acute gastroenteritis, which can cause severe diarrhoea and death if untreated.

■ **salpingitis**

inflammation of the fallopian tubes. See also **pelvic inflammatory disease.**

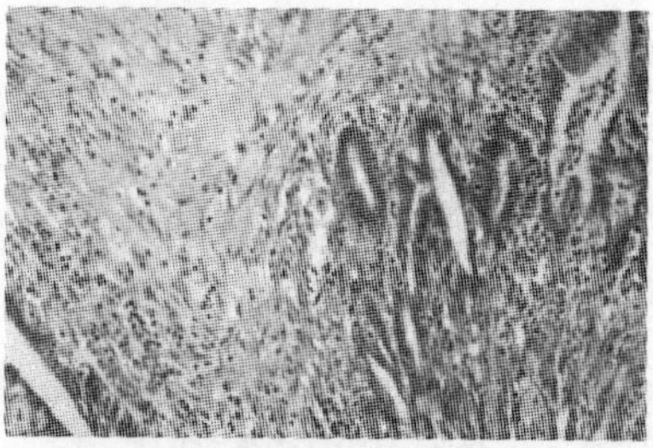

■ **salvage therapy**

emergency treatment with an experimental drug of an illness that has not responded to standard therapy.

■ **saquinavir (invirase)**

a protease inhibitor drug, the first in its class to be FDA-approved for the treatment of HIV disease. Current practice favours the use of saquinavir in combination therapy, e.g. with nucleoside analog drugs, to avoid the development of drug-resistant virus.

■ **sarcoma**

a malignant tumour of the skin or soft tissues.

■ **sc**

subcutaneous.

■ **scabies**

infection with the parasitic mite Sarcoptes scabieri, which causes an intensely itchy rash due to an inflammatory hypersensitivity reaction. Female mites burrow into the skin and lay eggs. The larvae live under the skin, causing the itching and rash. The rarer Norwegian scabies results in thick crusts on the skin. Scabies is highly contagious and may be transmitted by household or sexual contact. Infestation may be treated using an insecticide such as permethrin (Elimite) or lindane (Kwell).

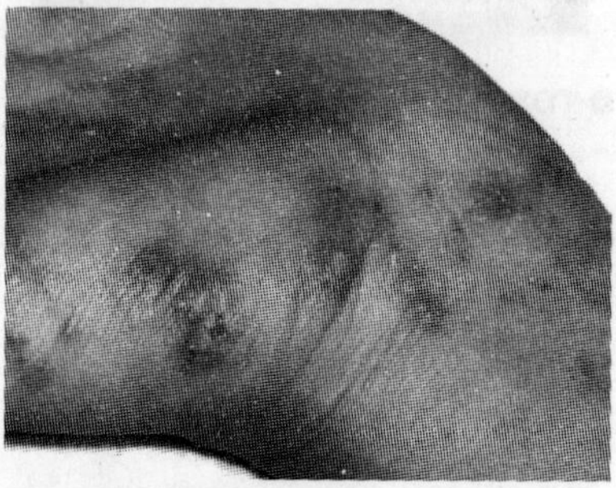

■ **scid mouse**

a mouse that lacks key immune system components. SCID mice are used as animal models in the study of transplantation and immune system disorders. SCID-hu mice have had their absent immune system replaced by human immune system components, allowing their use in the study of human immune disorders.

■ **sclerosis**
a hardening of tissue (e.g., liver, artery walls), due to cumulative damage, mineral deposition or other causes.

■ **scotoma**
area of blurred or reduced vision.

■ **scrotum**
the external pouch underneath the penis that contains the testes.

■ **scurvy**
a disease caused by a lack of vitamin C characterised by anemia and lesions of the skin and mucous membranes.

■ **seborrhea (seborrheic dermatitis)**
an overproduction of sebum by the sebaceous glands leading to an itchy red rash often accompanied by encrusted patches. Seborrhea typically occurs on the skin of the scalp, face, ears, chest or genitals. Seborrheic dermatitis is believed to be associated with a Pityrosporum fungus.

■ **secondary infection**
infection with a second or subsequent infectious organism during the course of an initial infection with another organism.

■ **secondary prophylaxis**
preventive treatment for a subsequent occurrence (relapse) of a disease. Contrast with primary prophylaxis.

■ **second-line treatment**
the second preferred therapy for a particular condition used when the patient fails or cannot tolerate the side effects of first-line treatment.

■ **Secretory Leukocyte Protease Inhibitor (SLPI)**
a protein found in saliva that binds to white blood cells and blocks HIV infection.

■ **sedative**
a drug that reduces mental activity and excitement.

■ **selenium**
a metallic trace element that combines with glutathione to form a major cellular antioxidant.

■ **senescence**
loss of function that accompanies aging.

■ **sensitivity**
the ability of an organism to be

affected by a drug or other agent. Sensitivity also refers to a statistical measure of the accuracy of a screening test, i.e., how likely a test is to label as positive those who have a disease or condition.

sensory ganglion (plural ganglia)
a cluster of nerve cells that connect the sensory periphery (skin, mucous membranes, muscle tissues, tendons, blood vessel walls, internal organ tissue) with the central nervous system.

sensory neuropathy
damage or necrosis of the sensory nerves, resulting in numbness, tingling or pain in the extremities. Sensory neuropathy is distinguishable from motor neuropathy, which may result in weakness and/or loss of motor coordination.

sepsis
the presence of pathogenic organism or their toxins in the blood or tissues. Symptoms include a sudden drop in blood pressure and changes in heart rate.

septic arthritis
infection in a joint.

septicemia
the physiological response to the presence of bacteria in the blood. Symptoms include increased cardiac and respiratory rates and fluctuations in body temperature.

sequelae
conditions resulting from a disease or injury.

seroconversion
the development of antibodies against a micro-organism. The change in a person's antibody status from negative to positive.

serology
the branch of medicine concerned with serum, the clear fluid portion of blood.

seronegative
having a blood test that does not indicate infection with a microorganism, either by the presence of antibodies or antigen.

seropositive
having a blood test result which indicates infection with an organism (e.g., HIV). A test may detect either antibodies to an organism (antibody positive) or the organism or its proteins (antigen positive).

seroreversion
the change in serostatus from positive to negative. Sero-reversion occurs in infants whose antibody status changes once they

have lost maternally transmitted antibodies.

■ **serostatus**

the presence or absence of an organism in the blood. Sero-status may be measured by the presence of antibodies against an organism (antibody status) or by the presence of the organism itself (antigen status). If antibodies or organisms are present, a person is said to be seropositive; if not, they are said to be seronegative.

■ **serotonin**

a neurotransmitter that has many effects, including blood vessel constriction and smooth muscle stimulation.

■ **serum**

the fluid, non-cellular portion of blood that remains after coagulation. The lymphatic fluid.

■ **Severe Combined Immunodeficiency (SCID)**

a condition, often genetic, in which more than one component of the immune system is compromised or dysfunctional, leaving an individual prone to a range of opportunistic illnesses and cancers.

■ **Sexually Transmitted Disease (STD)**

a disease that is transmitted through sexual contact.

■ **Serum Glutamic Pyruvic Transaminase (SGPT)**

see **transaminase.**

■ **shedding**

release of infectious particles (e.g., bacteria, viruses) into the environment, for example by sneezing, by foecal excretion or from an open lesion.

■ **shigellosis**

infection caused by Shigella bacteria. Shigellosis can cause digestive disturbances ranging from mild diarrhoea to severe dysentery.

■ **shingles**

see **herpes.**

■ **shock**

a condition characterised by the depression of mental and physical functioning, for example due to an injury or an allergic reaction.

■ **si**

syncytium-inducing strain of HIV.

■ **side effect**

adverse reaction. An allergic response to a drug. Some side effects are minor and others go away after a few days. A few are truly nasty and require quick medical attention.

■ **sigmoidoscopy**
examination of the sigmoid colon (the lower transverse part of the colon) with a lighted flexible viewing tube.

■ **sil**
see **squamous intraepithelial lesion.**

■ **Simian Immunodeficiency Virus (SIV)**
a viral infection endemic to African green monkeys and able to infect various primates. SIV is similar to HIV-2.

■ **single-agent therapy**
see **monotherapy.**

■ **sinus**
a hollow cavity. See also **paranasal sinuses.**

■ **sinusitis**
acute or chronic inflammation or infection of the paranasal sinuses (cavities behind the forehead and cheekbones), which may be characterised by nasal congestion and discharge, fever and headache. Sinusitis may be caused by bacteria, viruses or fungi or may be allergy-related. Treatment includes decongestants, antibiotics and surgical drainage.

■ **siv**
see **simian immunodeficiency virus.**

■ **sjögren's syndrome**
an autoimmune disorder characterised by dryness of the mucous membranes, enlarged salivary glands and facial lesions. The syndrome may also be associated with pancreatitis and kidney disease.

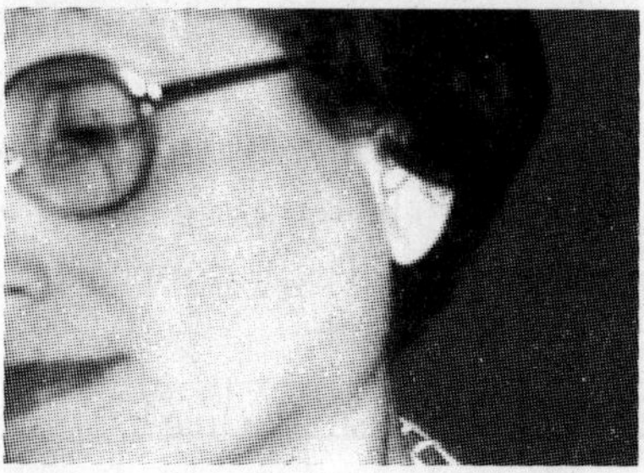

■ **slim disease**
a term for AIDS used in parts of Africa, so called because of the wasting effects of the disease.

■ **SLPI**
see secretory leukoctye protease inhibitor.

■ **sodium**
a trace element that is essential to many bodily processes including neural transmission.

■ **somatostatin (octreotide acetate)**
a pituitary hormone that inhibits the production of growth hormone and is used to treat diarrhoea.

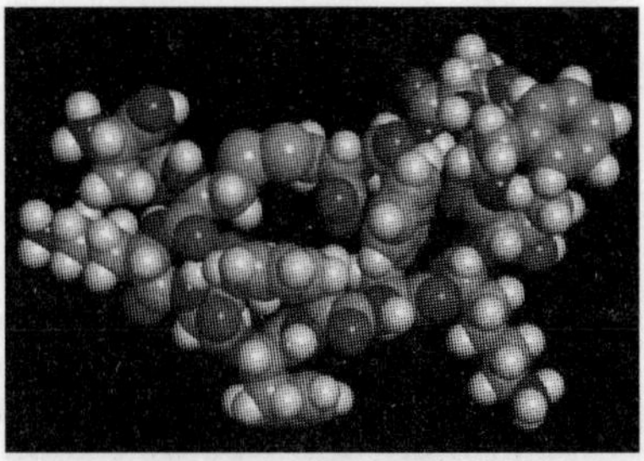

■ **somatotropin**
see **human growth hormone.**

■ **sorivudine (bv-ara-u)**
an antiviral drug used for the treatment of herpes simplex and varicella-zoster virus infection.

■ **spasticity**
a condition characterised by increased muscle tone, exaggerated reflexes and increased resistance to passive movement.

■ **specific immunity**
immunity directed against specific antigens. There are two types, TH1 or cellular and TH2 or humoral (antibody-based) immunity.

■ **speculum**
an instrument used to enlarge the opening of a canal or cavity (e.g., vagina, rectum, ear) in order to facilitate examination.

■ **spermicide**
an agent (e.g., Nonoxynol 9) that immobilises or kills spermatozoa. Spermicides are also often used to kill HIV and other organisms.

■ **sphincter**
a muscle that controls the opening of a duct or orifice, e.g. anal sphincter.

■ **spike**
a protein protrusion on the envelope of a virus. HIV spikes are composed of the glycoprotein gp120.

■ **spinal tap**
see **lumbar puncture.**

■ **spindle cell**
an unusually shaped cell found in Kaposi's sarcoma lesions.

■ **spirochete**
a class of bacteria that have a spiral or corkscrew-like appearance when seen under the microscope.

■ **spleen**
an organ of the lymphoid system located in the abdominal cavity. The spleen is a blood-producing organ in children and stores and disposes of red blood cells and platelets throughout life. The spleen is a reservoir for macrophages and is an important part of the immune system.

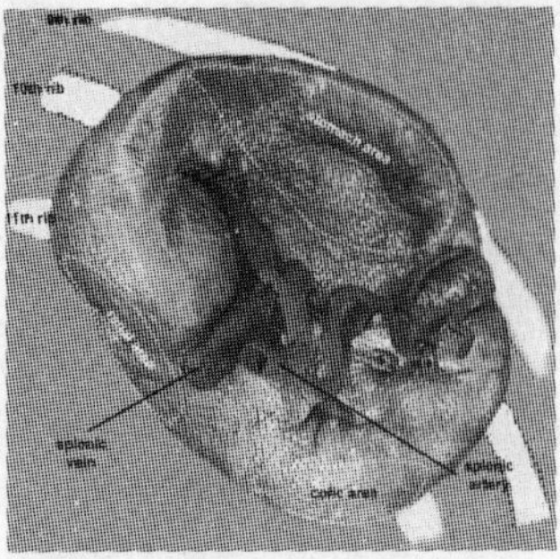

■ **splenectomy**
surgical removal of the spleen, which may leave the patient with a compromised immune system. Splenectomy may be performed to treat thrombocytopenia (low platelet levels).

■ **splenomegaly**
enlargement of the spleen.

■ **spore**
an early, latent reproductive stage of plants, fungi and some micro-organisms.

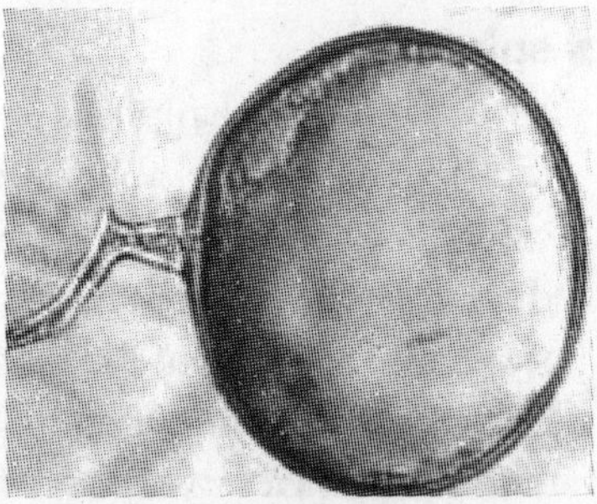

■ **sporotrichosis**
infection with Sporothrix schenckii, a diffuse cutaneous disease seen in immunocompromised people.

■ **sputum stain (sputum smear)**
a diagnostic test that uses mucus from the bronchial tubes.

■ **SPV-30**
a drug derived from the European boxwood tree that is under study as an anti-HIV therapy. SPV-30 may decrease levels of IL-2 and TNF-alpha.

■ **squamo-columnar junction**
the site where squamous cells lining mucous membranes meet columnar cells. Such an area is a common site for dysplasia.

■ **squamous cell**
a flat, thin cell that comprises the surface of the skin and the linings of the oesophagus, vagina and rectum.

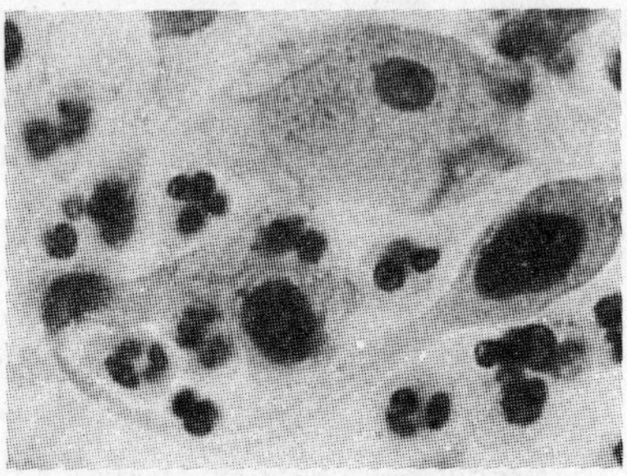

■ **Squamous Intraepithelial Lesion (SIL)**
abnormal growth of squamous cells. SIL particularly refers to ab-

normal cell changes at the squamo-columnar junction of the uterine cervix. Low-grade SIL is considered a precancerous condition.

■ ss

pharmaceutical abbreviation, one half (*semis*).

■ standard therapy

a therapy that is FDA-approved for a specific condition and is widely used as first-line treatment for that condition.

■ staphylococcus

a type of bacteria that cause various infections. Staphylococcus aureus is commonly present on the skin and mucous membranes, especially those of the nose and mouth. It can cause pus-containing lesions such as boils, carbuncles and abscesses. Other strains are associated with food poisoning and toxic shock syndrome.

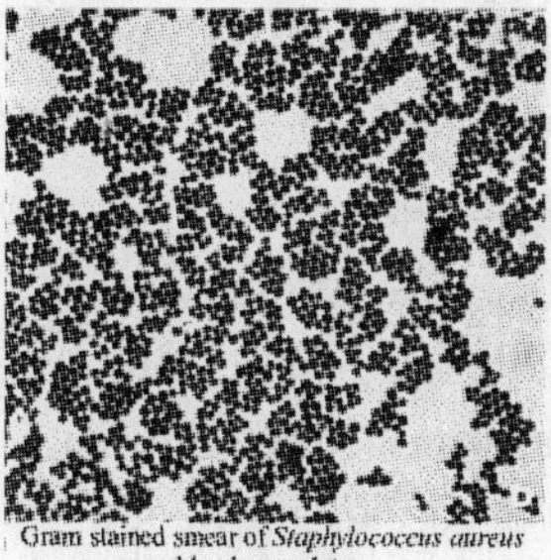

Gram stained smear of *Staphylococcus aureus* on blood agar plate

■ stat

pharmaceutical abbreviation, immediately (*statim*).

■ stavudine

see **d4T.**

■ STD

Sexually Transmitted Disease.

■ stem cell

a precursor cell from which blood cells are derived. As they mature, stem cells evolve into various types of red and white blood cells and platelets. Stem cells are located in the bone marrow, the site of blood cell production. Stem cells divide rapidly and are vulnerable to chemotherapy and radiation.

■ stenosis

narrowing or tightening of an opening or passage in the body.

■ sterility

inability to reproduce. Sterilisation is the process of surgically altering the reproductive organs as a permanent method of contraception.

■ steroid

a natural occuring compound (fat-soluble and having a 17-cargon-atom ring as a basis), including many hormones and vitamin precursors.

■ Stevens-Johnson Syndrome

an unusual, severe reaction

characterised by blistering and sloughing of the mucous membranes. The visceral organs may also be involved and the condition can be fatal. The syndrome may result from the use of certain medications such as TMP-SMX.

■ **stomatitis**
a swelling of the throat. This is an adverse reaction to some drugs, especially DDC.

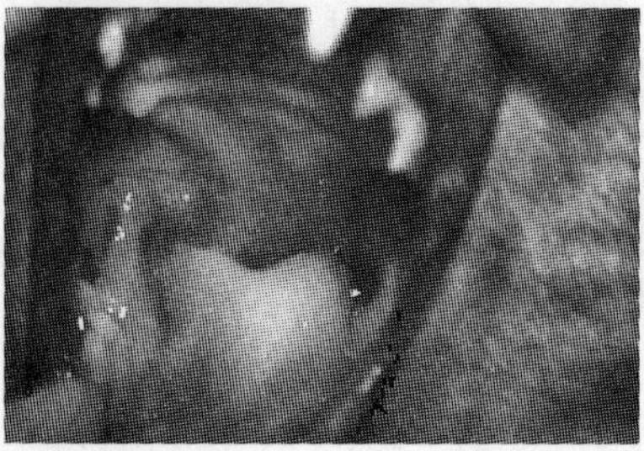

■ **strain**
a specific genetic variant of a particular organism. Many microorganisms have stronger and weaker strains, drug-sensitive and drug-resistant strains, etc.

■ **streptomycin**
an antibiotic used in combination therapy for tuberculosis and other infections. Side effects include nausea, dizziness, kidney toxicity and hearing loss.

■ **subclinical infection**
a low-grade asymptomatic infection.

■ **subcortical**
pertaining to structures in the interior of the brain. Subcortical dementia is a loss of mental, physical and/or emotional function due to organic disease of the brain's deep structures.

■ **subcutaneous**
an drug injection given just under the skin.

■ **sublingual**
under the tongue.

■ **subtype (clade)**
a phylogenetically distinct strain of a micro-organism. There are at least 11 subtypes of HIV-1 classified into 2 groups: group M (containing subtypes A through J) and group O. Subtype B is predominant in the U.S. There are 5 known subtypes of HIV-2 (A-E). See also **strain.**

■ **subunit**
a piece or small part of a larger unit.

■ **sulpha drug**
a class of sulphur-containing antibiotic drugs (e.g., sulfadiazine) which cause sensitivity or adverse reactions in many people.

■ **superantigen**
a viral or bacterial antigen that triggers an immune response

from a large number of immune cells (e.g., T-cells) which express a variety of different major histocompatibility (MHC) molecules.

■ superoxide dismutase

a naturally occurring cellular antioxidant that is part of the mechanism by which immune system cells kill or deactivate invading micro-organisms.

■ suppository

a tablet or troche that is inserted into the rectum or vagina.

■ suppression

the cessation of detectable viral replication in a person's blood.

■ suppressor T-cell

see **T-suppressor cell.**

■ surrogate marker

1.a marker or sign that can serve in place of a clinical endpoint such as the disease progression or death.

2.evidence of a condition. The most common HIV tests look for HIV antibodies instead of the actual virus. Those antibodies (or footprints) indicate the virus is present. Surrogate markers are used when they are easier to find than the actual organism.

■ susceptible

vulnerable to or potentially able to contract a disease, also refers to a micro-organism that is vulnerable to the effects of a drug.

■ sx

medical abbreviation for symptom.

■ symptom

1. a departure from normal function, sensation or appearance. A symptom is often an indication that a disease is present.
2.any perceptible change in the anatomy or function of the body that indicates the presence of a disease or condition.

■ syn-

prefix, together.

■ synapse

a small gap between neurons or between neurons and effector cells (e.g., muscle cells) where neural transmission takes places. Typically, a neurotransmitter is released into the gap (synapse) by a neuron and taken up by cells on the other side.

■ syncytium

a mass or clump of cells that fuse together to form one 'giant cell'. In HIV infection syncytium formation can lead to direct cell-to-cell infection. Strains of HIV are classified as either syncytium-inducing (SI) or non-syncytium-inducing (NSI). SI strains tend to infect T-cells, whereas NSI strains tend to infect macrophages.

■ syndrome

a set of symptoms or disease manifestations that occur together and characterize a specific condition.

■ synergism

the action of two or more substances to create an effect that none of the individual substances are capable of. For example, two drugs have synergism when one of the drugs makes the other drug more effective.

■ syngenic

transfer of blood or tissues from an individual with the same genotype (i.e., an identical twin). Contrast with allogenic.

■ syphilis

a sexually transmitted infectious disease caused by the spirochete bacterium Treponema pallidum. Stages of syphilis are primary (a nonpainful chancre in the mouth or anogenital area), secondary (a generalised rash, including the palms and soles, which occurs several weeks to a year later), a dormant stage in which the spirochetes remain in the body without causing symptoms and tertiary (which may affect many organs including the brain, leading to dementia [neurosyphilis] and death). In immunocompromised persons, syphilis may be progress more rapidly and be resistant to treatment. Penicillin is the usual treatment.

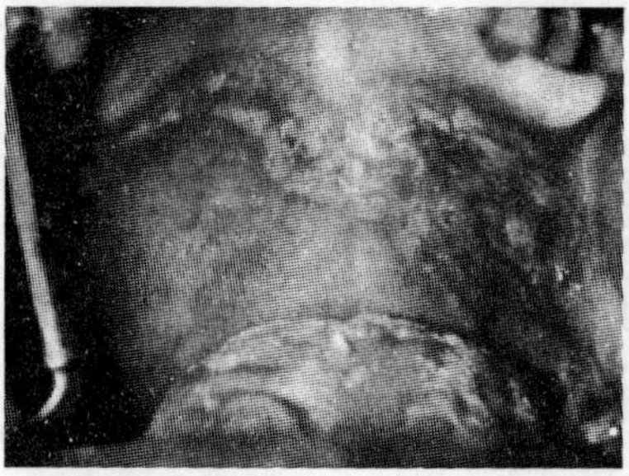

■ systemic

affecting the whole body. Contrast with localised.

■ systemic lupus erythematosus

an autoimmune disease of unknown cause characterised by swelling in many parts of the body, leading to blood vessel disorders, skin lesions, arthritis, nerve dysfunction and kidney dysfunction.

■ T cells

White blood cells that play an important part in the immune system. There are three different types of T cells, each of which has different subsets. The commonly measured T cells are helper T cells, killer T cells and suppressor T cells.

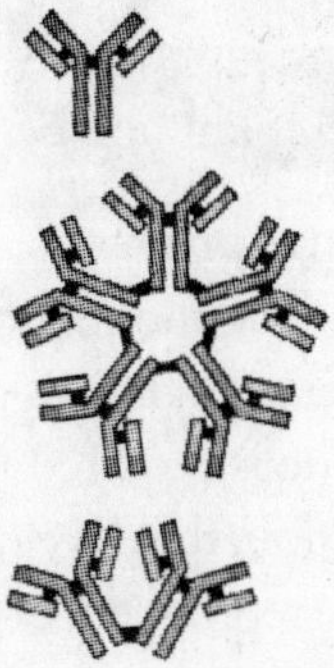

■ **T.I.D.**

pharmaceutical abbreviation, three times a day (*ter in die*).

■ **T.I.W.**

pharmaceutical abbreviation, three times a week.

■ **T4 cell**

see **CD4 cell.**

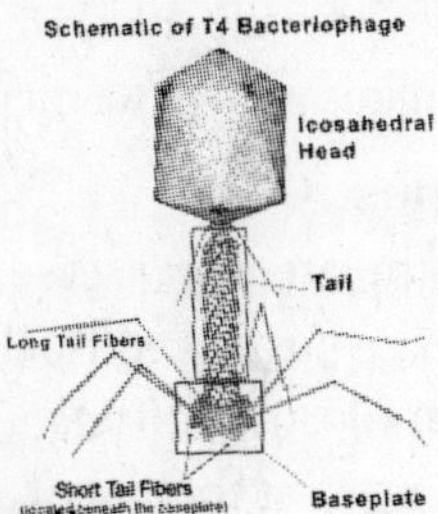

■ **T8 cell**

see **CD8 cell.**

■ **tachycardia**

very rapid heartbeat.

■ **tal**

pharmaceutical abbreviation, of such (*talis*).

■ **tat**

transactivator of transcription, a gene of HIV that plays a role in viral replication by regulating the transcription of viral DNA into RNA. Also the protein produced by that gene.

■ **tat inhibitor**

a drug that inhibits HIV replication by interfering with the tat protein.

■ **tb**

tuberculosis, a bacterial infection.

■ **T-cell (T-lymphocyte)**

a white blood cell derived from the thymus that contributes to the cell-mediated immune response. There are 3 major types of T-cells: T-helper (CD4 cells), T-suppressor (CD8 cells) and T-killer (cytotoxic T-lymphocytes or CTL). Contrast with B-cell.

■ **T-cell growth factor**

see **interleukin-2.**

■ **T-cell receptor**

a structure made up of several proteins located on the surface of T-cells. The receptor recognises antigens bound to major histocompatibility (MHC) molecules and triggers various cellular functions important to immune responses.

■ TCM

see **Traditional Chinese Medicine.**

■ telomere

a complex of repetitive DNA sequences that cap the ends of chromosomes. Telomeres play a role in cellular replication via the telomerase enzyme, which helps determine whether cells are able to replicate. Telomeres shorten each time a cell divides and signal cell senescence (loss of function) when they reach a critical length.

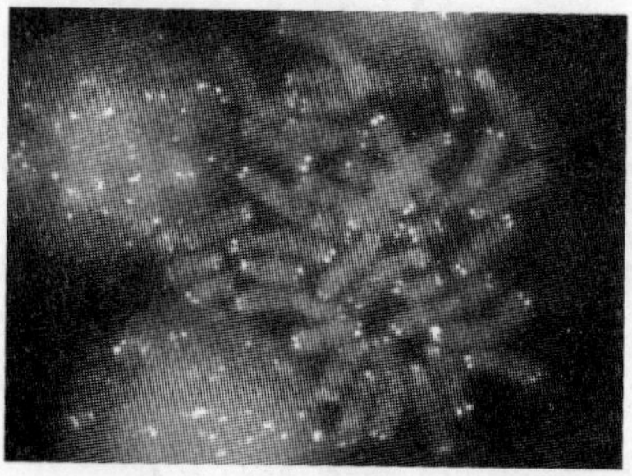

■ teratogenicity

the ability to cause malformation of the foetus (birth defects).

■ testis (testicle)

one of the male gonads located in the scrotal sac that are the site of sperm production.

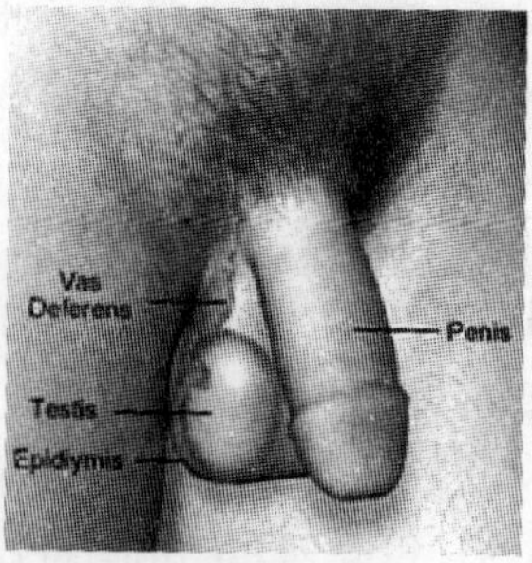

■ testosterone

a steroid hormone produced by the testes and adrenal glands. Testosterone is required for sperm production, the development of the male reproductive organs and the emergence of male secondary sexual characteristics. The hormone is also required for the build up of lean muscle mass. Testosterone levels are often low in HIV positive men. The hormone is under study as a therapy for wasting syndrome. Possible side effects include acne, mood swings, change in sex drive, liver toxicity, prostate enlargement and masculinisation in women.

■ tetanus

a life-threatening disease caused by toxins produced by the bacterium Clostridium tetani, which often grow at the site of a cut or wound. Muscles first become stiff, then rigidly fixed (lockjaw). Vaccination against tetanus should be done every 10 years or at the time of injury.

■ tetracycline

a broad spectrum antibiotic drug used to treat bacterial infections.

■ TH0 Response

an immune response that involves aspects of both TH1 and TH2 branches of the immune system. TH0 cells produce cytokines that are characteristic of both TH1 and TH2 response.

■ TH1 immune response

one of the branches of the immune system. The TH1 response involves a subset of CD4 lymphocytes, called TH1 cells that secrete IL-1, IL-2 and gamma interferon and which enhance the cell-mediated immune response (action of CTL and natural killer cells) and inhibit TH2 cell activity and the humoral immune response. TH1 activity is especially effective against agents that have infected cells, e.g. cell-associated HIV.

■ TH2 immune response

one of the branches of the immune system. The TH2 response involves the TH2 subset of CD4 cells that secrete IL-4 and IL-10 and which enhance humoral immune response (antibody production) and inhibit TH1 activity and cell-mediated immune response. TH2 activity is most effective against micro-organisms that are free-floating in the bloodstream, e.g. cell-free HIV.

■ thalamus

one of the basal ganglia (a cluster of nerve cell bodies) deep in the brain that serves as a centre for the relay of sensory information, especially pain and pleasure information and plays a role in arousal.

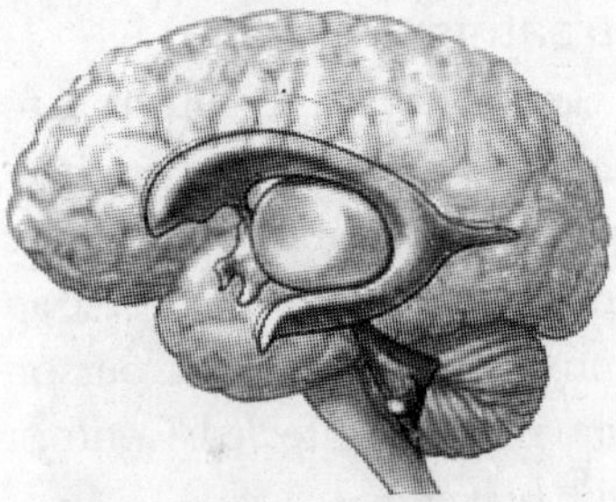

■ thalidomide

a sedative drug under investigation for treatment of aphthous ulcers, wasting syndrome and other conditions in persons with HIV disease. Thalidomide has been shown to reduce levels of tumour necrosis factor-alpha (TNF-alpha) in vitro. The drug has teratogenic effects and may cause severe birth defects. Other side effects include skin rashes and peripheral neuropathy.

■ **THC**
see **delta-9 tetrahydrocannabinol.**

■ **T-Helper Cell**
see **CD4 cell.**

■ **T-Helper Cell (T4 cell, Cd4 cell)**
a subset of T cells. Physicians regularly measure T-helper cell counts in HIV positive people. The normal range for T-helper cells is 480-1800, but may vary.

■ **therapeutic vaccine (treatment vaccine)**
a vaccine given after infection to reduce or arrest disease progression. Therapeutic vaccines are given to produce or reinforce an immune response in a person who is already infected. Contrast with preventive vaccine.

■ **therapeutic window (therapeutic ratio)**
the range of dosages of a drug that achieve clinical efficacy but do not cause intolerable side effects. The difference between the minimum and maximum effective doses.

■ **thiamine (vitamin B1)**
see **vitamin B.**

■ **thrombocyte (platelet)**
a type of blood cell that facilitates normal blood clotting.

■ **thrombocytopenia**
an abnormally low number of thrombocytes (platelets). The condition may result in abnormal bleeding and bruising. The normal platelet range is 150,000-300,000 per millimetre of blood. Thrombocytopenia may be controlled by the administration of certain cytokines or by removal of the spleen.

■ **thrombosis**
formation or presence of a clot within a blood vessel.

■ **thrush**
see **candidiasis.**

■ **thymic factor (thymic hormone)**
a hormone or cytokine (e.g., thymodulin, thymopentin, thymostimulin) produced by the thymus gland that is involved in the regulation of immune function.

■ **thymic humoral factor**
a peptide hormone isolated from calf thymus under study as an immunomodulatory treatment for HIV disease.

■ **thymidine kinase**
an enzyme that catalyses the transfer of phosphate groups and is necessary for the transformation

and metabolism of nucleoside analog drugs.

■ **Thymine (T)**
one of the pyrimidine nucleic acid bases that make up nucleotides, the building blocks of DNA (but not RNA). The antiviral drugs AZT and d4T are nucleoside analogs associated with thymine.

■ **thymus (adjective thymic)**
a lymphoid organ located in the chest behind the sternum. The thymus is a source of T-lymphocytes in children, but generally shrinks during adolescence. The thymus is the site of T-lymphocyte differentiation, where the cells learn to recognize antigens. The thymus produces some 30 hormones or thymic factors (e.g., thymodulin, thymopentin, thymostimulin) that are involved in the regulation of immune function.

■ **thyroid gland**
an organ at base of the neck that produces thyroxin and other hormones.

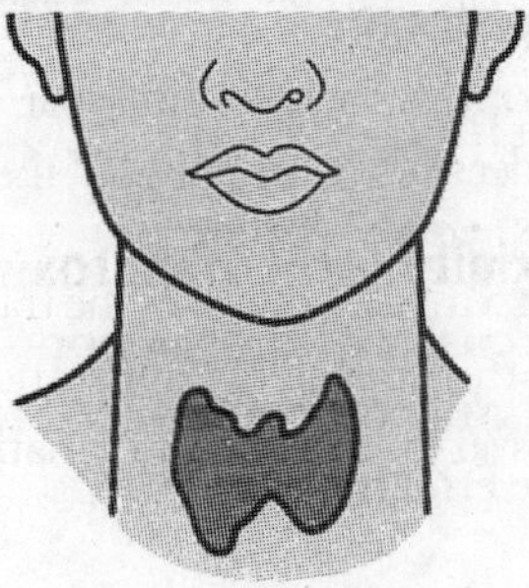

■ **Thyroid Stimulating Hormone (TSH)**
a pituitary hormone which stimulates the growth and function of the thyroid gland.

■ **TIBO derivative**
a synthetic compound derived from molecules similar to valium and related tranquilisers. TIBO derivatives have been shown to have potent anti-HIV-1 activity by blocking the production of reverse transcriptase.

■ **TID**
3 times per day.

■ **tincture**
a substance that colours, dyes or stains. Also refers to a medicinal preparation of an active ingredient or extract, e.g. of a plant dissolved in alcohol.

■ **tine test**
a skin test used to determine previous infection with tuberculosis. The tine test is an older test that has largely been superseded by the more accurate PPD test.

■ **tinea**
a group of infections of the skin, nails or hair caused by fungal organisms that typically cause a red, itchy rash. Types include tinea versicolor, tinea corporis (ringworm), tinea pedis (athlete's foot) and tinea cruris (jock itch).

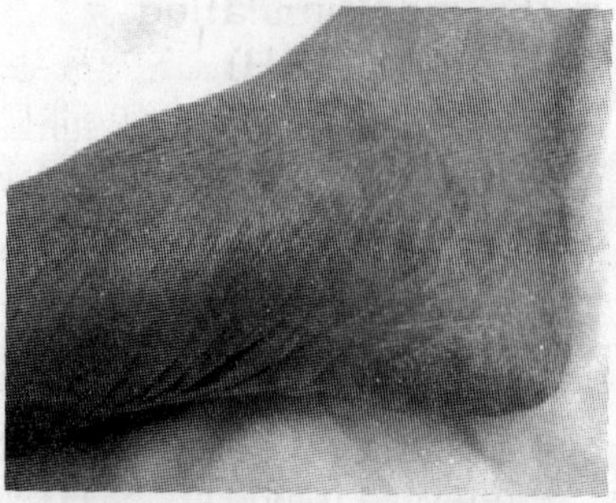

■ tinnitis

an abnormal ringing or buzzing in the ears. Tinnitis may be a side effect of certain medications.

■ titer (titre)

a standard measure of the strength or concentration of a component per volume of a solution.

■ titration

the measurement of volume; often used to refer to the determination of a drug dosage.

■ tiw

3 times per week.

■ T-killer cell (cytoxic t cells)

a type of white-blood cell that kills foreign organisms after being activated by T-helper cells.

■ tmp-smx

see **trimethoprimsulfamethoxazol.**

■ TNF (Tumour Necrosis Factor)

abbreviation, , a naturally occurring protein. TNF destroys cancer cells, but is suspected as being a co-factor in HIV replication.

■ tocopherol

see **vitamin E.**

■ tolerance

a condition in which the body becomes accustomed to an agent, e.g. drug so that the previous dose no longer produces the desired effects and a progressively larger dose is needed to achieve a previously observed effect. See also cross-tolerance.

■ tonsil

one of the 2 small immune system glands made up of lymphoid tissue, located at the back of the throat.

■ topical

pertaining to the surface of the skin. A medication applied to the skin.

■ topotecan

a topoisomerase inhibitor drug under study as an anti-HIV therapy.

■ toxicity (adjective toxic)

the quality of being poisonous or harmful; often used to refer to side effects of drugs.

■ **toxicology**
the study of the harmful effects of substances on the body, including the level of toxicity, the mechanism by which toxicity occurs and how it can be controlled.

■ **toxicosis**
a pathological condition resulting from poisoning.

■ **toxin**
a harmful or poisonous agent.

■ **toxoplasmic encephalitis (cerebral toxoplasmosis)**
see **toxoplasmosis.**

■ **toxoplasmosis (toxo)**
an opportunistic infection caused by the microscopic protozoan Toxoplasma gondii, found in undercooked meat and cat faeces. Symptoms may include headache, lymphadenopathy, malaise, muscle pain and fever. A common manifestation of the disease toxoplasmic encephalitis (cerebral toxoplasmosis), characterised by brain swelling, dementia, confusion, lethargy, seizures and coma; the eyes, heart and lungs may also be affected. Toxoplasmosis is treated with pyramethamine, usually in combination with other drugs; TMP-SMX may be used as prophylaxis.

■ **trace element**
a substance needed in very small amounts for the proper functioning of the body. There are 7 known trace elements: chromium, copper, cobalt, iodine, iron, selenium and zinc.

■ **trachea**
the windpipe, the tube that extends from the oral cavity into the chest, where it branches into the 2 major bronchial tubes.

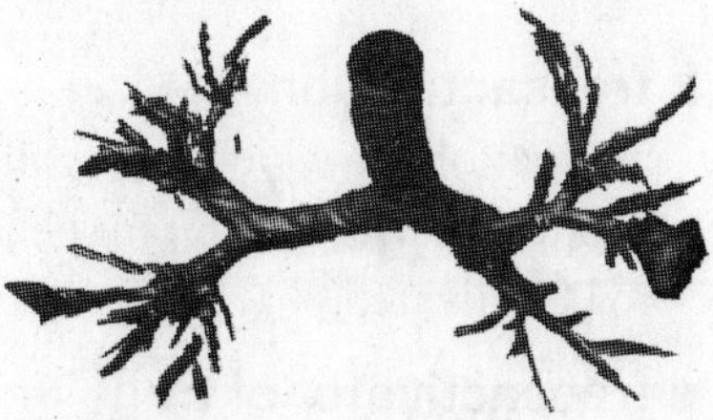

■ **tract**
an organ system that allows the body to interact with the outside world, e.g. gastrointestinal tract, respiratory tract. Also a bundle of nerve fibres, e.g. extrapyramidal tract.

■ **Traditional Chinese Medicine (TCM)**
an Asian system of healing that focuses on achieving internal balance. TCM practitioners use methods such as acupuncture, heat application (moxibustion),

herbal preparations and exercises (e.g., tai chi, qigong) to restore the flow of qi (vital energy) and the balance of yin and yang. TCM diagnosis is based on examination of the pulse and tongue. TCM diagnostic patterns typically seen in persons with HIV/AIDS are spleen qi deficiency, liver qi congestion, general qi deficiency and yin deficiency.

■ **trans-**
prefix, across, through or between.

■ **transactivation**
a situation in which one gene product causes a different gene to be activated.

■ **transactivator of transcription**
see **TAT.**

■ **transaminase**
an enzyme used as a catalyst in moving an amino acid from one compound to another. Doctors use a transaminase lab test to indicate liver function.

■ **transcription**
the first step in protein synthesis and replication. Genetic information encoded in DNA is copied to messenger RNA, which is used as a template for the production of new proteins.

■ **transcutaneous (transdermal)**
able to be absorbed by or to pass through intact skin.

■ **transdominant mutant**
genetically engineered, non-functional copies of HIV viral proteins that compete with functional HIV for the various molecules needed for viral replication.

■ **Transduced Autologous Fibroblasts (TAF)**
a type of gene therapy for HIV disease. Fibroblasts (collagen-producing cells) are removed from the body, genetically altered and re-infused into the body in an attempt to enhance the anti-HIV immune response.

■ **transduction**
the introduction of a transferred gene into a cell via genetic engineering techniques, e.g. a virus vector, liposomes.

■ **transfer factor**
a substance produced by white blood cells that transfers the ability to recognize foreign invaders from cell to cell.

■ **transformation zone**
the area of the cervix where squamous cells and columnar cells meet; a common site of dysplasia.

■ **transfusion**
the transfer of blood or blood components from one individual to another or back to the donor in the case of autologous transfusion.

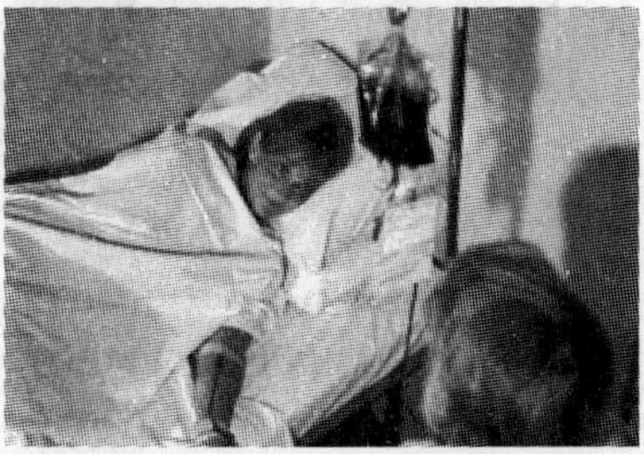

■ **transgenic**
pertaining to a chromosome or an organism into which genes from another individual have been inserted.

■ **transient**
short-lived; not permanent.

■ **treatment arm**
a group of participants in a research trial who all receive the same treatment. Contrast with control arm.

■ **Treatment Investigational New Drug (TIND)**
a FDA classification that allows physicians to prescribe certain promising experimental drugs prior to marketing approval for patients with life-threatening diseases who lack other treatment options.

■ **treatment vaccine**
see **therapeutic vaccine.**

■ **trental**
brand name of pentoxifylline.

■ **treponema pallidum**
the spiral-shaped bacteria that causes syphilis.

■ **tretinoin**
see **retinoic acid.**

■ **trial (study)**
an experiment involving the collection, analysis and interpretation of data, for example a clinical trial to determine the safety and efficacy of a new drug.

■ **triazole**
see **azole drug.**

■ **Trichomoniasis (TV)**
infection with the protozoan parasite Trichomonas vaginalis. Trichomoniasis may be asymptomatic, especially in men. In women, symptoms may include vaginal irritation, itching, discharge and painful urination.

■ **trichosanthin (compound q, glq223)**
the active ingredient derived from the root of the Chinese cucumber plant. Trichosanthin has been studied as an anti-HIV therapy and has been shown to kill HIV-infected macrophages. Side ef-

fects may be severe and include muscle and joint pain and central nervous system complications.

triglyceride
a combination of glycerol and fatty acids.

triglycerides
fat in the blood. A high triglyceride blood test can indicate liver or pancreas problems. A low result can indicate malnutrition.

trimester
a 3-month period; usually used to refer to one-third of the length of a normal human pregnancy.

Trimethoprim-Sulfamethoxazole (TMP-SMX)
an antibiotic drug combination. TMP-SMX is the preferred first-line therapy for prophylaxis and treatment of PCP and may be effective against other OI such as toxoplasmosis. Side effects include fever, nausea, diarrhoea, photosensitivity, skin rash and neutropenia. Desensitisation to the drug is often possible using slowly increasing dosages.

trimetrexate (neutrexin)
an antifolate drug used as salvage therapy for people with PCP who fail standard treatments. Trimetrexate can cause severe bone marrow toxicity and is typically used in conjunction with leucovorin to protect against anaemia.

trophoblast
the layer of cells covering the embryo that develops into the placenta.

tropism
affinity for or the tendency to move toward something; the specific attraction of a virus or other micro-organism to a particular host tissue, determined in part by host cell surface markers, e.g. some HIV strains have a tropism for CD4 cells.

trough level
the lowest concentration of a drug reached in the body between dosages.

T-suppressor cell
a type of T-cell bearing the CD8 surface marker. T-suppressor cells helps to regulate and control immune system activity by inhibiting antibody production and CTL activity.

tubal ligation
a method of permanent female sterilisation in which the fallopian tubes are cut.

■ **tubercle**
a granulomatous, spherical lesion containing a concentration of white blood cells, characteristic of infection with Mycobacterium tuberculosis.

■ **tuberculin reactive**
refers to someone who tests positive for exposure to tuberculosis on a PPD skin test.

■ **tuberculin skin test**
a skin test for exposure to tuberculosis. See **PPD test.**

■ **tuberculosis (tb)**
an infectious disease caused by Mycobacterium tuberculosis that typically affects the lungs, but may also occur in other organs (extrapulmonary TB). Transmission generally occurs through inhalation of aerosolised sputum droplets. A combination of 4 chemotherapeutic drugs is standard therapy. Multidrug-resistant tuberculosis (MDR-TB) is resistant to several standard drugs and requires more aggressive treatment.

■ **tubo-ovarian abscess**
a inflammation of the a fallopian tube and the companion ovary, characterised by swelling and accumulation of pus.

■ **tubule**
a small, narrow tube or anatomical channel.

■ **tumour**
a neoplasm, a new growth of rapidly proliferating cells. Tumours may be either benign or malignant (cancerous).

■ **tumour necrosis factor**
a naturally occurring protein, commonly called TNF. TNF destroys cancer cells, but is suspected as being a co-factor in HIV replication.

■ **Tumour Necrosis Factor (TNF, cachectin)**
a cytokine, produced by activated monocytes and macrophages, that can destroy tumours. When chronically elevated (as may occur in HIV disease), TNF-alpha may lead to fever, anorexia, hyper-metabolism and wasting. TNF-alpha may block the production of enzymes that digest fats, leading to the breakdown of muscle tissue. In laboratory tests TNF-alpha has been shown to stimulate HIV replication. Some drugs, e.g. thalidomide, ketotifen reduce TNF-alpha levels. TNF-beta is released by CD4 and CD8 T-cells when stimulated by an antigen.

tx

medical abbreviation for treatment.

tyrosine kinase

an enzyme that promotes various cellular processes by attaching phosphates to other molecules.

ubiquitous

widely present.

ulcer (ulceration)

an open sore of the skin or mucus membrane characterised by sloughing of inflamed dead tissue.

ultrasonography (ultrasound)

a method of visualising the internal parts of the body or a foetus within the uterus, using sound waves.

Ultraviolet (UV)

electromagnetic radiation beyond the violet end of the visible light spectrum. UV radiation induces tanning and sunburn of the skin and is associated with the development of skin cancer. UV is used to kill Mycobacterium tuberculosis in hospitals.

umbilical cord

the cord that connects the foetus to the maternal placenta, providing nutrients and removing wastes.

uncontrolled trial

a research study in which there are no participants taking a placebo or a alternate therapy. Contrast with controlled trial, placebo-controlled trial.

univariate analysis

a statistical analysis that considers only one factor or variable at a time. Contrast with multivariate analysis.

upregulation

an increase in the rate at which a process occurs, a substance is released, etc.

Uracil (U)

one of the pyrimidine nucleic acid bases that make up nucleotides, the building blocks of genetic material. Uracil takes the place of thymine (T) in RNA.

ureaplasma

a type of gram-negative bacteria found in the human genitourinary tract, throat and/or rectum. Ureaplasma may be sexually transmitted and is a cause of nongonococcal urethritis. Left untreated infection can lead to inflammation of the prostate in men and pelvic inflammatory disease in women.

■ **urethra**
the canal that carries urine from the bladder to the outside of the body.

■ **urethritis**
inflammation of the urethra.

■ **uric acid**
a substance found in the blood and urine that is a by-product of protein metabolism.

■ **urticaria**
itchy, raised, swollen areas on the skin or mucous membranes, often a manifestation of an allergic reaction.

■ **ut dict.**
pharmaceutical abbreviation, as directed (*ut dictum*).

■ **uterus**
the muscular pelvic organ of the female reproductive system in which the foetus develops. (*syn.* womb).

■ **uveitis**
an inflammation of the membranes (uvea) of the eye. Anterior uveitis is an inflammation of the frontal membranes, e.g. the iris and the choroid. The condition is characterised by pain and redness.

■ **v3 loop**
part of the gp120 envelope protein of HIV-1. The V3 loop is believed to triggers as strong antibody response and is the basis of several candidate anti-HIV vaccines, however, the region is extremely variable among HIV strains. (*syn.* v3 region).

■ **vaccination**
inoculation of a substance i.e. the vaccine into the body for the purpose of producing active immunity against a disease.

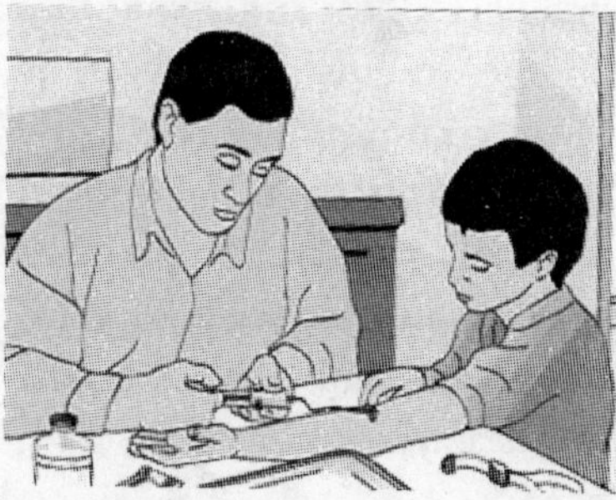

■ **vaccine**
a substance that contains antigenic components from an infectious micro-organism. By stimulating an immune response — but not the disease — it protects against subsequent infection by that organism. There can be preventive vaccines (e.g., measles or mumps) as well as therapeutic (treatment) vaccines.

■ **vaccinia**
a virus used as a vaccine against smallpox. Vaccinia is used as a live

virus vector is some candidate anti-HIV vaccines.

■ **vagina**

the passage from the uterus to the outside of the body, part of the female reproductive system; the 'birth canal'.

■ **vaginal candidiasis**

infection of the vagina and/or vulva with a yeast-like fungus, typically Candida albicans. Symptoms may include pain, itching, redness and a white discharge. Vaginal candidiasis is more common and more difficult to treat in HIV positive women; recurrent episodes may be an early sign of HIV infection. (vulvovaginal candidiasis, 'yeast infection').

■ **vaginitis**

inflammation of the vagina, often characterised by redness, irritation, itching and/or discharge. Vaginitis may be caused by a variety of factors, e.g. bacteria, Candida, hormonal changes.

■ **vaginosis**

see **bacterial vaginosis.**

■ **valacyclovir**

a prodrug of acyclovir used as an antiherpes treatment. Valacyclovir has significantly greater bio-availability than acyclovir and thus is effective at lower doses.

■ **varicella-zoster virus**

a herpes virus that initially causes chickenpox (varicella), usually in children. VZV may lie dormant within the nerves for years and reactivate later to cause herpes zoster (shingles), especially in immunosuppressed individuals. (VZV, human herpes virus 3).

■ **vascular hyperplasia**

excessive growth of the cells that form blood vessels, causing clusters of incomplete vessels in the skin or internal organs.

■ **vasculitis**

inflammation of the blood vessels.

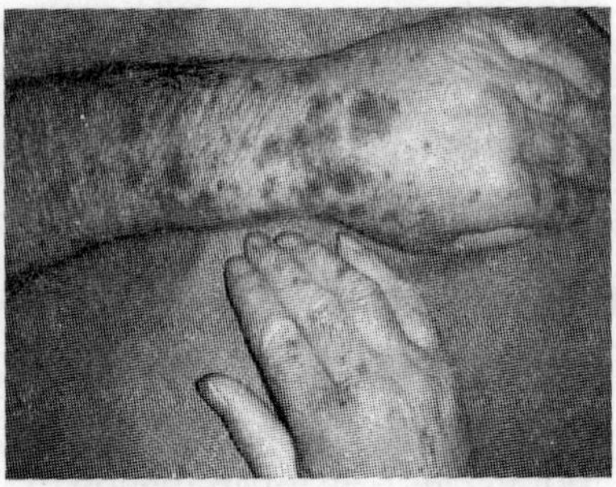

■ **vasodilation**

dilation of the blood vessels.

■ **vaxsyn**

a candidate anti-HIV vaccine based on the gp160 protein.

■ **VDRL Test**

Venereal Disease Research Laboratories test, a blood test for syphilis.

■ **vector**

an agent used as a vehicle for transfer. A disease vector is an agent that transfers a pathogen from one organism to another, e.g. an insect. A viral vector is an engineered virus used to introduce genes into cells or a live virus used as an antigen delivery vehicle in a vaccine.

■ **ventricle**

a partition, sac or cavity, e.g. the fluid-filled spaces in the centre of the brain, the chambers of the heart.

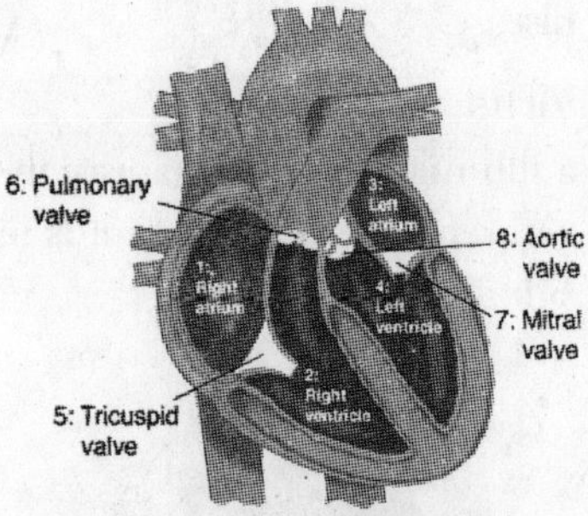

■ **vertical transmission**

transmission from a mother to a foetus or newborn. Vertical transmission may occur in utero (in the womb), intrapartum (during birth) or postpartum (via breast-feeding). Contrast with horizontal transmission. (perinatal transmission, mat).

■ **vertigo**

dizziness, a malfunction of the inner ear that makes the patient feel like everything is whirling around.

■ **VIF**

a gene of HIV, also the protein produced by that gene.

■ **villus**

finger-like projections of the intestinal wall that provide a large surface for the absorption of nutrients, *plural,* villi.

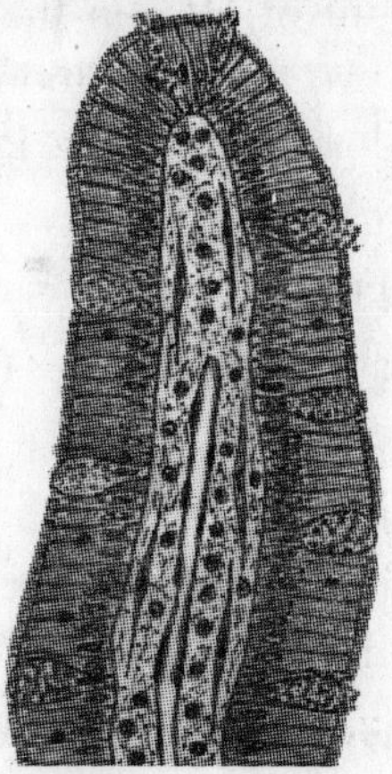

■ **vinblastine**

a chemotherapeutic drug used to treat various malignancies including Kaposi's sarcoma. Side effects include bone marrow suppression.

■ **vincristine**
a chemotherapeutic drug used to treat various neoplastic (cancerous) conditions including Kaposi's sarcoma and lymphoma. Side effects include peripheral neuropathy. (oncovin).

■ **violaceous**
purple.

■ **viracept**
brand name of nelfinavir.

■ **viral burden**
see **viral load.**

■ **viral load**
a group of tests that measure the amount of HIV in the blood. The two most commonly used viral load methods are PCR and bDNA.

■ **viral turnover**
the rate at which a virus dies and is regenerated.

■ **viremia**
the presence of virus in the blood.

■ **virilization**
development of mature masculine characteristics in a girl, woman or prepubescent boy.

■ **virion**
a complete virus particle that exists outside of a host cell.

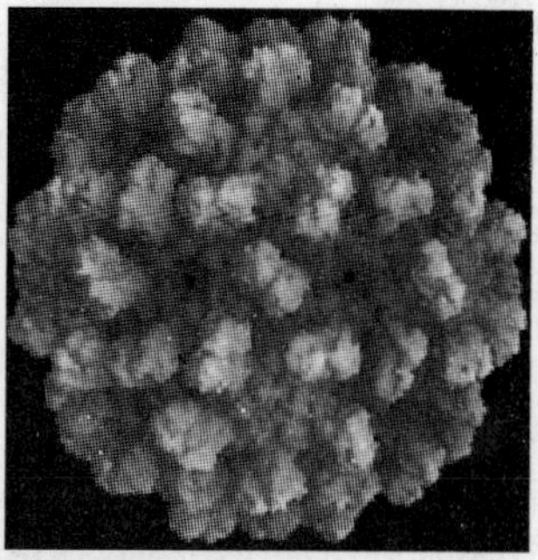

■ **virology**
the study of viruses and diseases caused by viruses.

■ **virucide**
a substance that can kill or destroy viruses. Contrast with virustatic.

■ **virulence (adjective virulent)**
aggressiveness, ability to cause disease.

■ **virus**
a sub-microscopic organism that can replicate only when it is inside another cell.

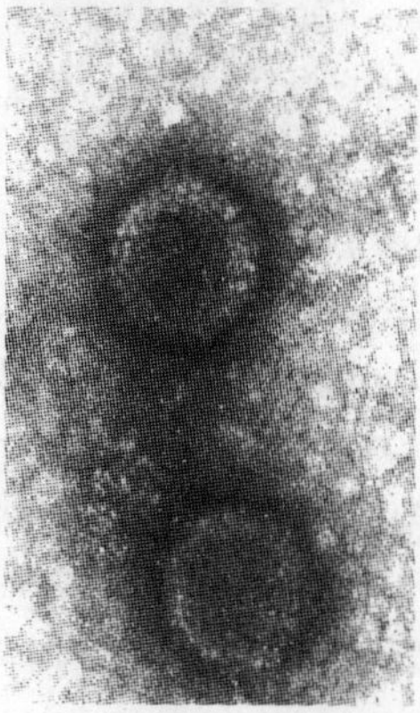

■ virustatic
a substance that has the ability to inhibit growth and/or reproduction of viruses without killing them. Contrast with virucide.

■ viscera (adjective visceral)
the major internal organs of the body (e.g., intestines, liver).

■ vistide
brand name of cidofovir.

■ vitamin
an organic substance that acts as a coenzyme and/or regulator of metabolic processes. There are 13 known vitamins, most of which are present in foods or supplements. Some are produced within the body. Vitamins are crucial for many bodily functions including a healthy immune response.

■ vitamin A
a fat-soluble vitamin with antioxidant properties that is essential for proper immune system functioning including lymphocyte development and maturation. Vitamin A deficiency is associated with impaired mucosal immunity and increased risk of vertical transmission of HIV. Excess vitamin A may be toxic to the liver. The vitamin is synthesised from beta carotene within the body.

■ vitamin B
a complex of several important vitamins including B1 (thiamin), B2 (riboflavin), B6 (pyridoxine), B12 (cobalamin). Vitamin B1 is needed for nerve signal transmission; deficiency may lead to neuropathy. Vitamin B2 is needed for the metabolism of amino acids; deficiency can result in eye and mouth pain and mental changes. Vitamin B6 is necessary for the production of many enzymes and chemical messengers (e.g., neurotransmitters); deficiency is linked to neuropathy and mental depression, skin rashes, nausea and seizures. Vitamin B12 is needed for red blood cell production and DNA synthesis and repair, deficiency may result in anaemia, neurological dysfunction, neuropathy and changes in mental status.

■ vitamin C (ascorbic acid, ascorbate)
an antioxidant vitamin that protects cells from oxidative damage. Vitamin C is necessary for the production of collagen (e.g., for wound healing), hormones and neurotransmitters; it may have a role in fighting infection. Deficiency results in poor healing, easy bruising and anaemia.

■ **vitamin D**
a vitamin that is important for mineral metabolism and which may play a role in immune function. Vitamin D is manufactured within the skin when exposed to sunlight. Deficiency is uncommon and may result in weak bones and kidney stones.

■ **vitamin E (Tocopherol)**
an antioxidant vitamin that protects cell membranes from oxidative damage. Deficiency is rare and may lead to peripheral neuropathy, poor balance and reduced reflexes. Alpha tocopherol and gamma tocopherol are 2 forms of the vitamin.

■ **vitamin K**
a fat-soluble vitamin, available in foods and manufactured by intestinal bacteria, that is essential for blood coagulation and important in certain energy transfer reactions.

■ **vitreous humour**
a transparent, colourless mass of soft, gelatinous material that fills the back portion of the eye, from the lens in front to the retina in back.

■ **vomcristine**
a chemotherapeutic drug used in the treatment of malignant conditions, (e.g., Kaposi's sarcoma, lymphoma).

■ **VPR**
a gene of HIV; also the protein produced by the VPR gene. The VPR protein is believed to play a role in HIV infectivity and pathogenesis.

■ **VPU**
a gene of HIV; also the protein produced by that gene.

■ **vulva**
the external female genitalia, including the clitoris and the inner and outer labia surrounding the urethral and vaginal openings.

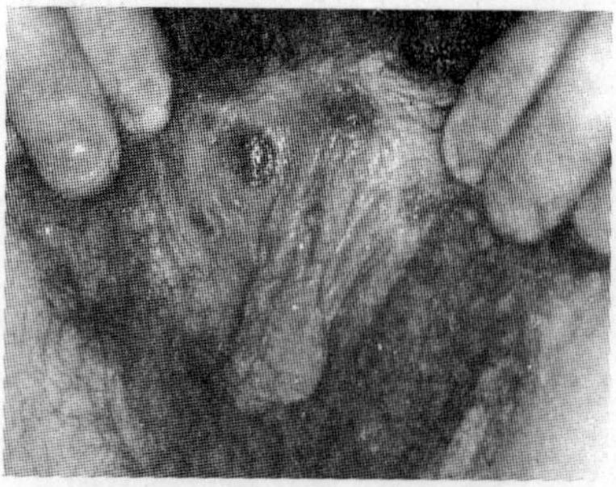

■ **vulvovaginal candidiasis**
see **vaginal candidiasis.**

■ **washout period**
the time it takes for a drug to be cleared from the body.

■ **wasting syndrome**
severe weight loss.

water soluble

capable of being dissolved in water. Water-soluble compounds are easily excreted by the body.

western blot

a laboratory test for specific antibodies to confirm repeatedly reactive results on the HIV ELISA or EIA tests. In the U.S., Western Blot is the validation test used most often for confirmation of these other tests. The Western blot uses an electrical field that separates out the various components by their molecular weight. This allows identification of antibodies to specific viral antigens, which show up as identifiable 'bands' on a strip of test paper.

wet mount

a type of laboratory test in which a sample of a body fluid is preserved on a slide and examined under a microscope for the presence of micro-organisms.

wheal

a welt; an elevation on the skin that may itch or burn, often characteristic of an allergic reaction.

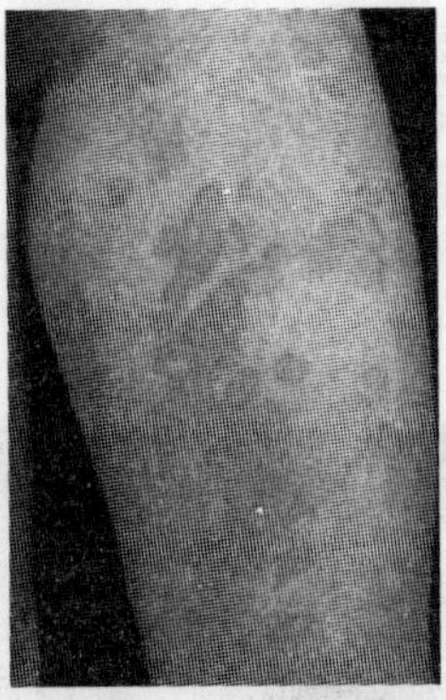

White Blood Cells (WBC)

part of the immune system, involved in fighting foreign substances. See **leukocyte.**

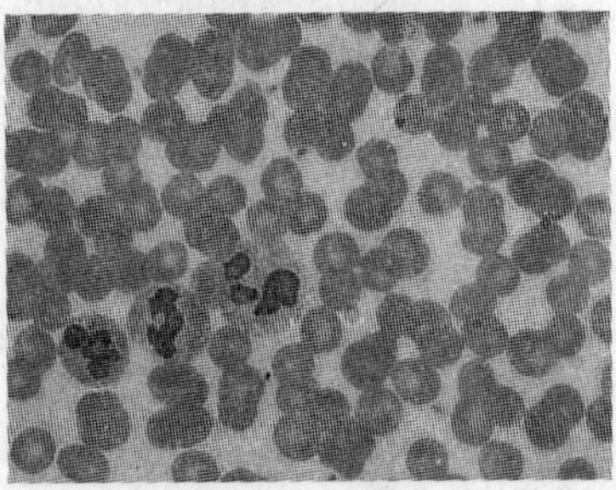

white matter

a type of neural tissue in the brain and spinal cord composed primarily of myelin-covered axons. Contrast with grey matter.

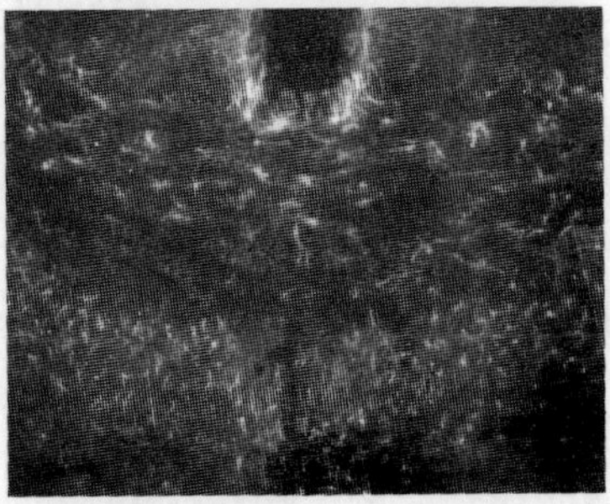

■ **whitlow**

an infection of the fingers caused by herpes simplex virus, usually the result of touching oral and/ or genital lesions.

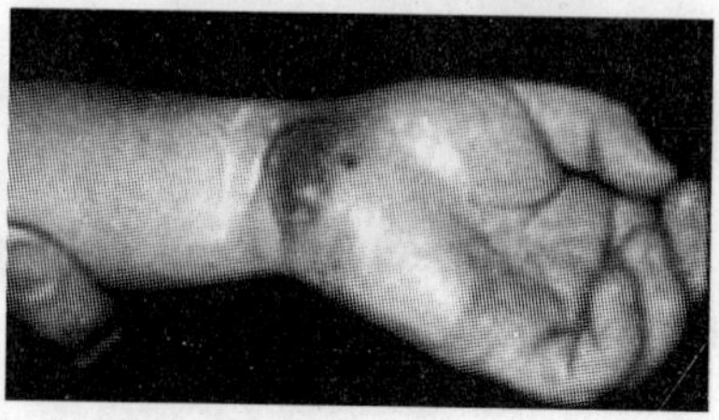

■ **whole-killed virus**

a type of vaccine in which a complete inactivated virus is used to provoke an immune response.

■ **WIHS**

abbreviation, Women's Interagency HIV Study. A multi-centre, prospective study, established in August 1993 to carry out comprehensive investigations of the impact of HIV infection in women. The rationale for establishing the WIHS was to investigate the clinical, laboratory and psychosocial aspects of HIV infection in women.

■ **wild-type**

the normal, typical phenotype of a virus or other organism before genetic mutation, manipulation or in vitro replication takes place.

■ **window period**

the time between primary infection and the appearance of antibodies against an organism (seroconversion).

■ **withdrawal**

a condition that results from the abrupt discontinuation of a dependency-inducing drug, characterised by symptoms such as sweating, tremors and nausea and pain.

■ **WNL**

pharmaceutical abbreviation, within normal limits.

■ **World Health Organisation (WHO)**

an organisation of the United Nations concerned with worldwide public health.

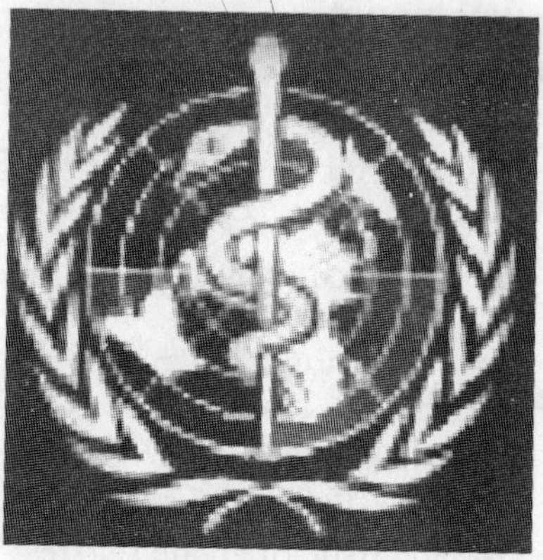

■ **yeast infection**

see **Candidiasis.**

■ **yeast infection**
see **vaginal candidiasis.**

■ **zinc fingers**
chains of amino acids found in cellular protein which bind to DNA or messenger RNA and play important roles in a cell's life cycle. They are called zinc fingers because they capture a zinc ion, which contributes to the array's binding to RNA or DNA. There are two zinc fingers in HIV's nucleocapsid. Zinc fingers are involved in binding and packaging viral RNA into new virions budding from an infected host's cell. The nucleocapsid protein and the zinc fingers also play a role during the process of reverse transcription. See **reverse transcription.**

■ **zinc finger inhibitors**
a class of experimental anti-HIV drugs which prevents the nucleocapsid part of the gag protein of HIV — which contains the zinc finger amino acid structures — from capturing and packaging new HIV genetic material into newly budding virons.
Miscellaneous

■ **µg**
pharmaceutical abbreviation, microgram.

■ **1592u89**
a nucleoside analog drug (see Abacavir and/or Ziagen).

■ **3tc**
a nucleoside analog drug that has fewer serious toxicities than other drugs of its class. 3TC has been approved in combination with AZT for the treatment of progressive HIV disease. Also called LAMIVUDINE, EPIVIR.

■ **5-fluorouracil (5-fu, effudex)**
a chemotherapeutic cream used to prevent and/or treat abnormal skin growths, neoplasias (especially cervical cancer) and warts.

■ **-emia**
suffix, the presence of a substance or component in the blood, e.g. viremia (presence of virus in the blood).

■ **-penia**
suffix, low levels or absence of a substance or component in the blood or serum (e.g., neutropenia indicates a low levels of neutrophils.

■ **-poiesis**
suffix, creation or formation, e.g. hematopoiesis is the formation of blood cells.

NOTES

34. Genetic Engineering	125/-
35. Health & Nutrition	125/-
36. History	125/-
37. Import and Export	125/-
38. Information System Management	125/-
39. Internet	125/-
40. IT	125/-
41. Inorganic Chemistry	125/-
42. Law	125/-
43. Library & Information Science	125/-
44. Literature	125/-
45. Management	125/-
46. Mathematics	125/-
47. Marketing & Sales	125/-
48. Mass Communication	125/-
49. Mechanical Engg.	125/-
50. Medical	125/-
51. Music	125/-
52. Organic Chemistry	125/-
53. Philosophy	125/-
54. Physical Education	125/-
55. Physics	125/-
56. Psychology	125/-
57. Science	125/-
58. Sex	125/-
59. Sociology	125/-
60. Sports	125/-
61. Textile	125/-
62. Zoology	125/-